T0392271

Applied Drama and Person-Centred Nursing

Karl Tizzard-Kleister

Applied Drama and Person-Centred Nursing

How drama can enhance the education and performance of person-centred practice

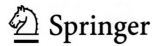 Springer

Karl Tizzard-Kleister
Health Action Training Ltd.
Derry/Londonderry, UK

ISBN 978-3-031-77207-8   ISBN 978-3-031-77208-5   (eBook)
https://doi.org/10.1007/978-3-031-77208-5

© The Editor(s) (if applicable) and The Author(s), under exclusive license to Springer Nature Switzerland AG 2024
This work is subject to copyright. All rights are solely and exclusively licensed by the Publisher, whether the whole or part of the material is concerned, specifically the rights of translation, reprinting, reuse of illustrations, recitation, broadcasting, reproduction on microfilms or in any other physical way, and transmission or information storage and retrieval, electronic adaptation, computer software, or by similar or dissimilar methodology now known or hereafter developed.
The use of general descriptive names, registered names, trademarks, service marks, etc. in this publication does not imply, even in the absence of a specific statement, that such names are exempt from the relevant protective laws and regulations and therefore free for general use.
The publisher, the authors and the editors are safe to assume that the advice and information in this book are believed to be true and accurate at the date of publication. Neither the publisher nor the authors or the editors give a warranty, expressed or implied, with respect to the material contained herein or for any errors or omissions that may have been made. The publisher remains neutral with regard to jurisdictional claims in published maps and institutional affiliations.

This Springer imprint is published by the registered company Springer Nature Switzerland AG
The registered company address is: Gewerbestrasse 11, 6330 Cham, Switzerland

If disposing of this product, please recycle the paper.

This book is dedicated to nurses around the world who work to save our lives and to make them better. If this book helps one person to start or continue to do that, then I count it as a massive success.

I also dedicate this book to my late Grandmothers, Shirley Kleister and Rose Tizzard. Though I miss them both, their lessons on how to care deeply, to persevere through adversity, and to always see the uniqueness in people continue to live with me.

Foreword

It is an honour and a pleasure to write the foreword for this book, which makes a significant contribution to the evidence base on person-centred nursing, through the use of applied drama. Karl is a researcher who has had the courage to navigate the interdisciplinary research space, which is not without its challenges, particularly when bridging two distinctly different disciplines. The account of his work in this book is eloquently written, with a passion for his practice and for making a difference. As such, this is a book that will appeal to a wide audience, ranging from researchers to practitioners, to educators, and to students across both fields of practice.

Person-centredness is recognised as the fundamental philosophical positioning for healthcare globally, and the reason—simply stated—is that respecting the humanity of people really matters across our healthcare systems. It prioritises the human experience and places compassion, dignity, and humanistic caring principles at the centre of planning and decision-making and is translated through relationships that are built on effective interpersonal processes. Despite this, person-centredness has been the subject of much discussion and debate, having been heralded as too difficult to define and challenging to implement in busy practice environments. Yet, we continue to uncover failures in our systems that have long-lasting impacts on patients, families, carers, and healthcare practitioners. The kind of work described in this book is at the forefront of preparing student nurses to embody the values of person-centredness and be able to enact that in practice, thus preparing them to be role models and champions for person-centredness, but more importantly, system leaders for the future.

The person-centred nursing framework is the underpinning theoretical framework used in Karl's research, which was originally developed as a means of operationalising person-centred nursing practice. The framework is recognised as a mid-range theory that shines a light on practice and brings a shared understanding and a common language to person-centredness in nursing. As the authors of the framework, we welcome new insights into the components of the framework through robust research such as this, which enhances our understanding and increases the potential to make a greater impact.

A key focus of this book is on being sympathetically present, one of the five person-centred nursing processes presented in the person-centred nursing framework. This process describes 'an engagement that recognises the uniqueness and value of the person, by appropriately responding to cues that maximise coping resources through the recognition of important agendas in their life' (McCormack and McCance 2021: p. 19). This is one of the most contested person-centred processes, with challenges levied at the use of the term sympathy as opposed to empathy. Karl's work makes a significant contribution to evidencing the importance of this process and how it characterises being present in the moment, influencing the quality of person-centred interactions. In Chap. 2, he undertakes a critique of the contemporary literature on empathy, challenging its dominance through the lens of sympathetic presence. From this position, Karl's work aims to explore, understand, and discover if there is a potential relation between drama-based approaches to learning and the development of practical skills in person-centred nursing—specifically the process of sympathetic presence.

Key findings are beautifully storied in Part 2 of this book, taking the reader through stages that include: moving from self-centredness to person-centredness; overcoming vulnerability; attending to others; and finally, to performing presence. What is elucidated is how a sympathetic presence is the first position in approaching interactions, which enhances the other person-centred nursing processes. This is an example of how we can bring the invisible to life: it can be difficult to explain sympathetic presence using words or even thinking about it—thinking about it is much easier after you have experienced it (McCance et al. 2021).

Finally, Karl's book provides insights into the interdisciplinary exchange between the fields of drama and nursing, focusing on the impact on nursing education through drama-based facilitation approaches. His contribution aligns with our goals for person-centredness in the curriculum and the creativity required to 'teach' students about being person-centred. Engaging in critical and creative methods such as drama and dramatic representation enables us to embody key person-centred practices, including being sympathetically present. We know that moving our understanding from our heads to our hearts enables key practices and processes to become embodied and more likely to be normalised in our daily ways of being and doing—what Angie Titchen refers to as the 'professional artistry' of practice (Titchen 2009). Professional artistry is difficult to put into words because it is deeply embodied and embedded in our praxis. It is never possible to completely articulate the complexity of the professional artistry of person-centred practice, because it is deeply embodied in our personhood. However, the methods and practices developed by Karl through his scholarly inquiry go a long way towards helping us to articulate the essences of the professional artistry of person-centred practice. Karl's drama practice that is so successful in articulating this essence reminds us of a line from the Brian Friel play 'Dancing at Lughnasa':

> *Dance as if language had surrendered to movement – as if this ritual, this wordless ceremony, was now the way to speak, to whisper private and sacred things, to be in touch with some otherness … Dancing as if language no longer existed because words were no longer necessary*

References

McCormack B, McCance T (2021) The Person-centred nursing framework. In: Dewing J, McCormack B, McCance T (eds) Person-centred nursing research: methodology, methods and outcomes. Springer, New York, pp.13–27

McCance T, McCormack B, Tizzard-Kleister K, Wallace L (2021) Being sympathetically present. In: McCormack B, McCance T, Bulley C, Brown D, McMillan A, Martin S (eds) Fundamentals of Person-centred healthcare practice. Oxford, Wiley-Blackwell, pp 139–146

Titchen A (2009) Developing expertise through nurturing professional artistry in the workplace. In: Hardy S, Titchen A, McCormack B, Manley K (eds) Revealing nursing expertise through practitioner inquiry. Wiley-Blackwell, Oxford, pp 219–243

Ulster University
Belfast, Northern Ireland

University of Sydney
Sydney, NSW, Australia

Tanya McCance

Brendan McCormack

Preface

Situating This Study

This book will explore approaches within the crossover of applied drama and person-centred nursing (PCN), synthesising practices and concepts to develop a unique approach to nursing education and lighting a path to understanding what person-centred facilitation (PCF) could be. This book is firmly rooted in the research I undertook during my PhD studies at Ulster University, which to the best of my knowledge is the only PhD to date that has been jointly awarded by a school of nursing and a school of drama. The majority of the perspectives in this book are rooted in the geographical context of the United Kingdom (UK) and from my experience and heuristic as a white, British, middle-class (with working-class roots), heterosexual, male. I am no fan of labels and their overuse, much preferring the notion of personhood—and thus identity—to be something co-constructed in the moment and in relation to oneself and others. I prefer fluidity to essentialism and relationality to fundamentalism. However, I acknowledge the importance of positioning aspects of my personhood, which have and continue to influence my perspective and approach to my life and the tremendous impact this has had and continues to have on my research. I contend that it is vital not to attempt to remove oneself from one's work for three main reasons. First, this is almost impossible; second, doing so means that important elements of the work can be over-generalised; and third, doing so can remove the vitality of character that I can bring to my work. I hope that this book will not only involve the notion of applying drama to PCN and vice versa but also of applying personhood and person-centredness to research.

Londonderry, UK   Karl Tizzard-Kleister

Acknowledgements

I would like to extend my gratitude to the many people who have supported me in reaching this point.

First, I would like to acknowledge my PhD supervisors, Tanya McCance, Matt Jennings, and Brendan McCormack. It is their confidence in me that has instilled in me the confidence to undertake the PhD and subsequently write this book. My PhD journey, like that of many others, was often challenging. Their patience and guidance helped me navigate the most challenging parts. Their critical friendship continues to challenge me to flourish. All three have been mentors to me, not just in how to be a good academic but also in how to be a good person too.

I am deeply grateful to Tanya and Brendan for their generosity in writing a wonderful foreword for this book; I genuinely could not think of a better seal of approval for my work than their endorsement.

I would also like to extend my gratitude to Pat Deeny for the delight with which he readily shares his expertise and experience and for his warmth and kindness. I consider it a privilege to call him my friend.

I owe a huge debt of gratitude to Prof. Jenny Moore, who so kindly offered her expertise and editorial support as this book neared completion. Your insights played a crucial role in getting this book over the line.

Another thank you to the folks at Springer for their interest in my work, and their support and patience whilst I slowly pieced it together.

A heartfelt thank you is extended to my colleagues at Health Action Training, who are a joy to work with, as well as to all the wonderful people who have joined our sessions since our inception in May 2020. Many of the insights I have gleaned, a large amount of which can be found in this book, have come from the work we have done together.

The last few thank-yous are reserved for my family. First, to my father, Steven Tizzard, who has always encouraged me to think differently about the world. He worked as a care professional and taught me what caring for others truly meant—that it is not just about completing a 'task', but always doing what is right to make people's lives better. Second, to my mother, Wanda Kleister, for the love and support she has always given me, no matter what, and for making me the person I am today. I have heard that a 30-second hug with another person releases endorphins, making us feel good—if that is the case, I have 30 years' worth of endorphins to thank her for.

Lastly, my wonderful partner, Kayleigh Nunn. Thank you for making my life full of joy and for teaching me how to be utterly comfortable just being me. I am so grateful for you.

Contents

Abbreviations

ACE	Arts Council England
ACI	Arts Council Ireland
APPG	All-Party Parliamentary Group
CPR	Creative personal reflections
DRACAR	Drama caring and reflection in nursing education
EM	Emotion memory
GMC	General Medical Council
MoPA	Method of Physical Action
NHS	National Health Service
NMC	Nursing and Midwifery Council
OSCE	Objective structured clinical examination
PCC	Patient Client Council
PCN	Person-centred nursing
PCF	Person-centred facilitation
PCNF	Person-centred nursing framework
PCP	Person-centred practice
PCPF	Person-centred practice framework
RCN	Royal College of Nursing
SRP	Simulated role play
TIE	Theatre in education
TNA	The National Archives
TO	Theatre of the Oppressed
UU	Ulster University
UK	United Kingdom
WHO	World Health Organization

Introduction

1

Introduction

This chapter will introduce the fields of drama and nursing. It will explore immediate crossovers to lay the groundwork for the rest of the book in terms of developing a joined conceptual framework. Following that, I will consider the contemporary moment, present a case study based on my doctoral study that will serve as a touchstone throughout the book, address some key distinctions and features of how the disciplines of drama and nursing view evidence, and finally—following a person-centred approach—I will present a positioning of myself as a researcher and practitioner engaged in this study.

Drama and Nursing: Addressing Interdisciplinarity

Into and throughout the 2010s, there was a growing interest in how drama and performance relate to notions of care, health, healthcare, and well-being (White 2009; Brodzinski 2010; Baxter and Low 2017). Entering the early 2020s, this interest swelled, alongside the rapid rise of arts and health[1] as an increasingly significant field of study. In contemporary studies and practices, drama is acknowledged as an approach that enhances nursing education (Mermikides 2020; Arveklev et al. 2020; Kyle et al. 2023). This book aims to add to the growth of this particular movement in a very specific way. This book seeks to address the insights to be gained when exploring the interdisciplinary exchange between the fields of drama and nursing,

---

[1] Throughout this book, I use the term 'arts and health' as a catch-all term. There are important debates around the distinctions between terms like 'arts and health', 'arts in health', 'arts for health', 'art and medicine', 'health humanities', and so on. For ease of reading, I will use 'arts and health' as a chosen catch-all, meaning any intersections between arts and health in the broadest sense.

© The Author(s), under exclusive license to Springer Nature
Switzerland AG 2024
K. Tizzard-Kleister, *Applied Drama and Person-Centred Nursing*,
https://doi.org/10.1007/978-3-031-77208-5_1

focusing on the impact on nursing education through the development of particular drama-based facilitation approaches.

Arguably, drama[2] is amongst the least considered art forms explored in the field of arts and health. For instance, Fancourt's seminal text *Arts in Health* (2017) only mentions drama briefly and only provides a few examples of organisations that use drama in health contexts. Another example is found in the equally seminal collection from Clift & Camic, *Creative arts, health, and wellbeing* (2016) where, though drama is mentioned frequently, no chapter focuses solely on drama as a central topic, whereas multiple chapters highlight music, visual arts, and dance. Finally, this can be seen in the 2017 All Party Parliamentary Group (APPG) report *Creative Health* which in the United Kingdom (UK) served as a flash point for the field of arts and health. When conducting a simple key term search of the document, it has far less mention of drama (20 instances) or theatre (41) than, for example, music (326) and dance (176). This is not to say that drama does not have a clear and defined place within the field of arts and health, but that the lower level of attention highlights the need for more attention on drama and health, and more exploration of discrete art forms more broadly in the arts and health. Moreover, it speaks to the need to acknowledge the difference that applying drama to healthcare specifically has when compared to other art forms, such as music or dance.

Similar to how drama is perhaps less considered in the field of arts and health, nursing has traditionally been seen as subordinate to medicine and, though this view has been challenged in modern times, the working relationship between nurses and medics is still evolving and is often contentious (Mohammad et al. 2022). PCN, in particular, challenges the power dynamic between nursing and medicine and seeks to resist the standardisation and mechanisation through the over-medicalisation of the nursing profession (McCormack and McCance 2010). Often PCN can be seen as a shift from nursing as a primarily technical approach to one that is also a moral and ethical practice striving for the rights of each person and their health (Smith 2016). Nursing is also arguably under-considered in the field of arts and health, especially compared again to medicine. Returning to the example of representation in seminal texts on Arts and Health, only one chapter in Clift and Camic's (2016) collection focuses specifically on nursing.[3] Considering also that the medical humanities constitute something of an entire subfield within arts and health, and there is currently no established field of 'nursing humanities' (though, see Damsgaard 2020 for advances in that area), nursing can be argued to be

---

[2] Again, throughout this book, I am using the term 'drama' to mean the dramatic arts more broadly. This includes drama, theatre, applied drama, performance, community drama, and so on. There are some points in this book where specific terms are given and explored (see Chap. 2's exploration of the term 'applied drama'), but otherwise the term 'drama' will serve as a catch-all term.

[3] See Noonan et al. (2016) in Clift and Camic (2016). It is worth mentioning that nursing is of course mentioned elsewhere in that collection, the point I am making is not that nursing is ignored, but that considering that nurses comprise the largest proportion of healthcare professionals in many healthcare systems (see statistics in the UK context here: The healthcare workforce across the UK—Office for National Statistics (ons.gov.uk)), only having one chapter dedicated to nursing may suggest nursing is under-represented in the literature on arts and health.

under-represented in arts and health. This book aims to address the under-representation of drama and nursing in the fields of arts and health and champions the need for specificity within interdisciplinary work. As such, the two specific areas this book explores are applied drama and PCN. At times broader points are raised, but this should always be understood through the prism of the intersection between applied drama and PCN.

As a field arts and health has a predilection towards generalisable outcomes, where the main drive seems to be to build a repository of evidence that adds to a central argument; that engaging in creative approaches is good for us. This is an admirable aim, and the argument is thankfully becoming one that is difficult to argue against (APPG 2017; Fancourt and Finn 2019; Fancourt et al. 2020). However, the desire from arts and health researchers to build an evidence base to support that statement as an overwhelming concern means we may miss out on specific, complex, and detailed outcomes—as well as crucial contextual factors for why art is important, and why that particular art for that particular person may be helpful (Vickhoff 2023). It is my experience as a researcher straddling the 'divide' between nursing and drama that having clear and specific aims and using specific methods in conjunction across disciplines is the major strength of the approach. I also wish to highlight specificity and criticality to avoid the assumption that participation in the arts is always good for you.

It is not too early in this text to offer a firmly held position I have constructed throughout the development of the book: the arts and health researchers who do not welcome, embrace, and translate practices and principles from disciplines outside of their main area are not engaging in true interdisciplinarity. Doing so ring-fences their discipline from the potential gains from mutual exchange across disciplines. This is not to say that researchers should be uncritical of practices and principles transferring across other disciplines and their own. Rather, they should recognise that they are seeing from their disciplinary perspective. They must make an active effort to attend to their disciplinary biases, embrace disciplinary differences, and find a way to translate between these differences. This is an under-considered and difficult feature of such work and a largely invisible act of labour undertaken by an interdisciplinary researcher. This study will explore this as a feature throughout, and I hope to affirm that generosity is the defining feature of the admirable interdisciplinary researcher, who shares, adapts, and translates practices and principles to make disciplinary boundaries less like bold lines, and more like blurred edges. The first step for this book's aim to blur the edge between applied drama and PCN is to deliberately smudge the line between them.

Blurring the Edge

The practices and principles of nursing have long been associated with kindness, respect, and compassion (Nursing and Midwifery Council (NMC) 2015, 2018). Nursing pedagogy promotes these attributes as necessary for 'person-centred' practice. McCormack & McCance, in the Person-Centred Practice Framework (PCPF), identify the importance of 'respecting the patient's rights as a person, building mutual trust and understanding and developing therapeutic relationships' (2016: p. 1). Meanwhile, applied drama and associated drama-based areas have become influenced by similar ideas. Recent developments in applied drama and health have focused on care ethics and aesthetics. The field of applied drama has found resonance with relational ethics of care, such as described by Gilligan (1990), Held (2006), Tronto (2013), and Noddings (2013), amongst many others. As such, attention from applied drama scholars has turned towards aesthetics found in relationships and care practices involved in applied drama processes. This area has been termed the 'aesthetics of care' (Thompson 2015, 2023; Nicholson 2017; Stuart Fisher and Thompson 2020). It is in this purposefully blurred intersection between Person-Centred Nursing (PCN) and applied drama that this book sits, where caring practices are measured by their aesthetics and their capacity for therapeutic and humanistic relationships, whilst the artistry and aesthetics of performance are entangled with the notion of care. This study needs to be distinguished from the medical humanities, which aims to humanise medicine. PCN needs no such humanisation, as it is an explicitly humanistic approach (Jacobs 2015; Jacobs et al. 2017), particularly in its roots from Rogers (1961) and Kitwood (1997) amongst others. This study has the specific aim of applying interactive drama-based education to PCN conceptually and practically, to enliven and embody what it means to perform person-centredness, and finally to build an approach that can add to PCN's capacity to resist depersonalisation found in some healthcare education and practice.

Some suggestions for applying PCN approaches have been successful in healthcare environments, and Person-Centred Practice (PCP) is espoused by organisations such as the World Health Organisation (WHO). However, 'evidence continues to show that far from humanising healthcare, people receiving healthcare continue to have mixed or poor experiences' (Dewing et al. 2017: p. 21). Ideas like those explored in the PCPF, as well as the Person-Centred Nursing Framework (PCNF) (McCormack and McCance 2006; Dewing et al. 2021), might be mostly considered theoretically, with less focus on how these constructs can be applied in practice. This reflects how others have identified significant gaps between theory and practice in nursing, which drama-based approaches might help to bridge (Ekebergh et al. 2004; Yakhforoshha et al. 2017). To address the perceived gap between nursing theory and practice, this book aims to explore how drama has already addressed this and suggest ways it might continue to do so. Along with exploring practices and approaches across the globe, this book will focus on a particular example, namely my doctoral study.

This book is based on work conducted during my doctoral studies, with much of the book drawn directly from my doctoral thesis. For clarity, the element that serves as a direct case study within this book is the primary research I conducted for my PhD. To briefly summarise, my primary research involved designing and delivering a series of drama-based workshops with a cohort of undergraduate nursing students. Though this whole book is indeed a result of my doctoral study, at times I may discuss this piece of primary research directly, and when doing so will refer to it as 'my PhD/doctoral study', or something along those lines. This is to delineate that primary research from the broader study that is this book. A central aim of my PhD was the creation of a bespoke drama-based course underpinned by concepts from the PCNF, and the implementation of this course with undergraduate nursing students. This book will return to this PhD study as a central case study pivotal in addressing the question of how drama might enhance a practical understanding of PCN constructs expressed through the PCNF.

In Part 1, the 'background' research is explored, including the outcomes from reviewing the literature and a construction of what a shared conceptual framing for PCN and applied drama might be. Part 2 is where the results of the PhD study are discussed concerning the ideas developed in Part 1. Before this, I will give some attention to the term 'sympathetic presence', as it proved to be a central concept from the start through to the very end of the study.

Conceptual Groundwork: (Re)Defining Sympathetic Presence

As it is a key concept for this study, there is a need to lay robust groundwork for the term sympathetic presence. This includes acknowledging and understanding the definitions of the term from PCN developed from 2006 onwards (McCormack and McCance 2010, 2016; McCormack et al. 2021) as well as positioning the term in context with drama-based theories and practices. Therefore, it is necessary to present an overview of the term early on in this book. This includes its origins, applications, and resonances with drama. This is intended to facilitate further exploration of the term throughout this book. It is no surprise that, amongst all of the factors, terms, and processes in the PCNF, sympathetic presence found a foothold for me in the process of applying drama to PCN. Sympathetic presence can be articulated as the main person-centred process in which we are immediately present with other persons. A characteristic of drama is the creation of moments and environments in which we encounter others, both a physical immediate presence and a theoretical one that asks us to engage with the perspectives of those embroiled within the drama at play. For me, sympathetic presence is fundamentally a dramatic process. As this book will explore, this does not mean dramatic in the sense of, say, a high drama or a melodrama. Instead, it involves the performance of presence, dialogue between persons and bodies, and an appreciation for the role one's own self has in engaging with others; three concepts that I contend are commonly found in drama.

Sympathetic presence is 'an engagement that recognises the uniqueness and value of the individual, by appropriately responding to cues that maximise coping resources through the recognition of important agendas in their life' (McCormack and McCance 2016: p. 102). When sympathetically present the nurse is 'in the moment' (McCormack and McCance 2010: p. 104), paying attention to how other people feel, without trying to assume or share their emotional or physical state. McCance et al. (2021) explore how the process of sympathetic presence is a way to bridge the theories of person-centredness with a practical application. Sympathetic presence as it is defined and how it has come to be understood describes an embodied presence characterised by sympathy (McCormack and McCance 2010, 2016). I suggest sympathetic presence is a process through which person-centeredness is actualised. It is enhanced through knowing the other person, and requires a skill set in recognising and often validating what others present as their personhood in a given moment. As McCance et al. (2021) summarise, it is 'more than just being physically present [...] [i]t is an openness and connection with the other person, which is emotional, cognitive, rational, and, at appropriate times, physical' (p. 141).

Sympathetic Presence and PCN as a Conscious Move Away from Empathy

Empathy, though often seen as a virtuous concept, has seen criticism for perpetuating stereotypes, encouraging discrimination, leading to burnout, and more (Kirk 2007; Cunico et al. 2012; Bloom 2018). Moreover, developing empathy in healthcare students has proven to be problematic (Hojat 2009; Nunes et al. 2011; Brodzinski 2014). Klimecky et al. (2014) describe a project exploring how empathy training can be damaging for healthcare professionals, where they feel compelled to vicariously experience the feelings of others in distress. They argue for compassion as an antidote, exploring how focusing on our will to help others rather than trying to fully understand the suffering of others is a better long term focus for professionals. Hojat (2009) theorises sympathy and empathy as overlapping processes, with compassion at their intersection. Others, such as Jeffrey (2017), criticise empathy as an individualistic concept and practice, and argue for an approach which is more relational. As such, to move from empathy to compassion, we must perhaps practice more sympathy and relationality. McCormack and McCance (2010) would certainly advocate for this, particularly through their term sympathetic presence.

The term has been heavily scrutinised and at times criticised. The majority of criticism revolves on the perception of sympathy as pity, meanwhile many suggest empathy is superior and more applicable for nursing and healthcare. Perhaps oversimplifying, sympathy suggests a 'feeling for' others and empathy a 'feeling with' others. It is not hard to see how sympathy can be seen as promoting pity, and how empathy can be helpful when caring for others. However, as McCance et al. (2021) suggest by drawing on the work of Wasylko and Stickley (2003), Mearns and Thorne (2007), Williams and Stickley (2010), and Hojat (2009), empathy requires us to be able to 'accurately perceive' another person's feelings (McCance et al. 2021: p. 142). Though we may be able to come close to understanding the unique experiences and emotions of others, we cannot fully understand their perspective, and so I argue empathy is not possible (McCormack and McCance 2016). It can also be said to run counter to person-centredness as a humanist philosophy (Rogers 1961; Kitwood 1997), where we assume we know what another person is experiencing and are less attentive to their perspective as a result. This is particularly relevant in healthcare contexts, where professionals can easily assume they understand what those in care are going through, and so instead of listening they rush to do what they think is right without considering the unique needs of those they wish to help.

Jennings et al. (2020) highlights how 'some attempts to improve empathy within nursing education have been counterproductive' (p. 192). For example, Ward et al. (2012) found that healthcare students reported lower empathy scores after their studies. The reason for this decline was unclear and the study raised more questions than it was able to answer, clearly paving the way for future research. The authors discuss many possible reasons why they and many other researchers in similar studies found an empathy decline in a variety of healthcare students. They highlight teaching methods in undergraduate nursing in particular as a strong potential factor. They summarise that 'many of these teaching methods favour efficiency over the fostering of human connectedness' (ibid, p. 38). Meanwhile, a study by Heggestad et al. (2016: p. 793) discovered that undergraduate nursing students appeared to suppress their responses to challenging clinical situations, through what Storaker et al. (2017) call 'emotional immunisation'. Student responses became increasingly limited to the realm of 'cognitive empathy', which as Heggestad et al explain is 'the capacity to understand and imagine the lived experiences of other persons' (2016: p. 787). 'Cognitive empathy' specifically describes understanding another person through thought, logic, and reasoning. This is often with the aid of imagination, but exclusively through cognition rather than feeling or embodiment. It can be linked to certain aspects of emotional intelligence, perspective-taking, and so on. Cognitive empathy is often seen in contrast to 'affective empathy', which Heggestad et al describe as 'both a bodily and spontaneous emotional experience' (Ibid). 'Affective empathy' can be described as feelings experienced and embodied in response to, and aligned with, the feelings of others. These students, perhaps understandably, were better prepared to consider another person's situation through rational understanding, rather than allowing themselves an emotional reaction to the feelings of another person. What can be implied here is that little to no attention is given to nursing students on the skill and practice of balancing between affective and cognitive empathy—or in more evocative terms, balancing between listening to the heart and the head when trying to understand and engage with others.

As Jennings et al. (2020) point out, 'practitioners who resist or reject affective empathy might be trying to manage the demands of the emotional labour of care (Hochschild 1983; Smith 1992)' (Jennings et al. 2020: p. 193) Though not unconsidered, the demand to manage the emotional labour of nursing could certainly be given more attention. For example, in the NMC (2018) standards of practice document, there is no mention of the term 'emotional labour', and no direct acknowledgement that nurses need to consider and recognise emotions and vulnerabilities in themselves as well as patients. Nnate and Nashwan (2023) discuss the effects of not acknowledging the impact of emotional labour in challenging communication scenarios for nurses, such as breaking bad news. They suggest that emotional intelligence should be a key consideration for frameworks and approaches to these tricky encounters. Inadvertently, by acknowledging that empathy can make it hard for nurses to 'detach themselves from the patient's experience' (p. 3), whilst assuming its usefulness for nursing practice, Nnate & Nashwan provide an argument that emotional intelligence serves as a buffer for nurses to the ill effects of over-empathising. It could be argued the issues surrounding empathy seen by the studies described above may be the result of a tactic on the part of nursing students to avoid emotional burnout. This is tempered by the possibility that the only option student nurses might feel they have is to try to immunise themselves against the pain of others they encounter. Heggestad et al. (2016) observes that although 'affective empathy' may be desirable in some situations, students can often experience 'empathic overarousal'. Empathetic overarousal is Hoffman's (2000) term, explaining when 'affectivity becomes so overwhelming that it becomes uncontrollable for the person and clouds his or her judgments' (Heggestad et al. 2016: p. 792). This observation connects to the PCNFs critique of empathy. Empathy is certainly not evil, but I argue it is often misunderstood, and when many of us use the term, we do not mean empathy, but something like it. This is why a key feature of my book is championing specificity, as many might find the distinction between sympathetic presence and empathy esoteric. I hope to present a strong argument for how being specific on the difference between these processes can light a path to developing Person-Centred Practitioners and/or Person-Centred Facilitators (PCF). Both terms are useful, yes, but assuming empathy is wholly good clouds the fact that it is not suitable to use in many contexts, it is in these contexts that we should turn to sympathetic presence.

Putting these findings of the potential pitfalls of empathy as a practice in a contemporary cultural, social, and political moment points towards the precarious moment we find ourselves in. Namely, these pitfalls have been exacerbated by the long-running systemic devaluation of both fields of exploration within this book, and the fallout from a global pandemic.[4] Switching gears from the academic to the cultural/political shines a spotlight on the state of both disciplines. Over the last 40 years, Drama has seen 'diminishing development' in curricula (Readman 2023). Meanwhile, drama and performance have been callously cut from curricula (Neelands et al. 2015), and the place of creative arts in schools is turbulent (see: 'Creativity crisis' looms for English schools due to arts cuts, says Labour | Arts in schools | The Guardian), whilst many drama organisations have had their funding pulled away like a tablecloth whipped out by a wicked flick of the wrist in what is being called a national emergency (see: 'A national emergency': UK theatres fear closure after more local funding cuts | Arts funding | The Guardian). As a result of these cuts politicians and policymakers after the challenges faced by the arts during the COVID-19 pandemic crassly painted a career in the arts as non-desirable with an advert advocating for ballet dancers to consider moving into the IT professions (see: Government scraps ballet dancer reskilling ad criticised as 'crass'|Culture|The Guardian).

Likewise, Nursing has faced incredible pressure. In 2015, it was announced that bursaries to study nursing were going to be scrapped (see: Why were nurse bursaries removed?—The Health Foundation), leading to shortfalls in recruitment to nursing degrees. Organisations such as the RCN are advocating for nursing 'beyond a

---

[4] I am mostly speaking about the UK context here, but this is certainly not an isolated phenomenon—where the dramatic arts are amongst the first cuts made by policymakers, for many different reasons and often under the dual guise of money saving as well as pragmatic thinking. In simple terms, the dramatic arts are presented as expensive, and serving no 'purpose'.

bursary' and rightly highlighting that though the bursaries are not a 'cash cow' for students, they ascribe a clear value and worth to the profession (see: Looking beyond the bursary|RCN Bulletin|Royal College of Nursing). Recently, bursaries for nursing studies have been brought back though offered as a fraction of what they were [see: Student nurses will get £5000 grant from next year as ministers battle to hire 50,000 more NHS nurses (inews.co.uk)]. Funding cuts across the National Health Service (NHS) place continued demand on all staff and services (see: Warning over cuts to NHS services without £10bn extra funding—BBC News), leaving over a quarter of registered nurses facing hardship [see: Nurses' cost of living: More than a quarter face hardship (personneltoday.com)] and record numbers of nurses leaving the profession [see: The NHS nursing workforce—have the floodgates opened?|The King's Fund (kingsfund.org.uk)]. Far more importantly—speaking from the standpoint of the COVID-19 pandemic—nurses have lost their lives to protect and save the lives of others. Less readily recognised, and just as important, is how nurses have worked extremely hard, applied immense expertise, and lost their lives to ease the passing of the lives of others, who have no other comfort than the presence of nurses and their fellow healthcare workers.

Seeing empathy as the only solution in these contexts is at best callous, and at worst a tactic of repression. This book and the reconfiguration from empathy to sympathetic presence offers a pathway for supporting nurses, through the expertise of drama professionals. This project calls for an enlivening relationship between, what can rightly be called, oppressed groups to find new ways of engaging with and caring for others, and ourselves. In clear terms, I am arguing for an interdisciplinary approach where nurses can develop crucial and practical skillsets in interaction and person-centredness, whilst applied drama practitioners can learn new—person-centred—ways of working with people who desperately need support. I also argue both disciplines can ill afford a reliance on empathy as a sustained approach. In short, seeing empathy as the only option is contributing to the drastic burnout of nurses, and drama professionals working through PCN may offer some approaches to challenge and change that, in so doing highlighting the immense value drama can have, and thereby highlighting its place in our society.[5]

---

[5] As an artist now working in an applied context, I am always drawn to the argument of 'art for art's sake'. Hopefully, I can address elements of this argument with the concepts at play here throughout this book. Though it is worth stating clearly at this point that I am sceptical of the statement that art should be for art's sake alone. Dismissing the potential impact that the arts can make is—I believe—negligent to its potential, and (as I will explain more later) an elitist position which ring fences arts practice and appreciation. I don't mean to suggest all art should serve a distinct and utilitarian purpose, nor that such purpose should be applied like a sticky label onto work to serve a goal such as securing funding. In short, I am arguing for—and echoing Thompson (2023)—art that cares.

Resonances with Drama, Empathy as Coercive

As Jennings et al. (2020) state, 'political and applied theatre artists have rejected the perception that drama should generate empathy through identification with a hero, as originally suggested by Aristotle' since the early twentieth century (p. 193). Influential theatre practitioners and theorists such as Brecht (1978) and Boal (1998) have urged a move away from traditional storytelling and theatre's reliance on empathy. Their main criticism of empathy is how it is coercive, and how when partnered with theatre it can be used to manipulate people and reduce their independence as well as capacity for communal action. As Nicholson (2005) explains, applied drama is rooted in criticisms like these, where rather than feeling with a protagonist and experiencing moments of catharsis, we use drama to reflect on the world and practice the creation of a better one. As Jennings et al. (2020) summarises, applied drama calls for 'dramatic forms that encourage critical discourse and pragmatic community action; for theatre that supports actual social change' (p. 193). They continue on this path to illustrate how this shift from empathy to more active and relational forms in theatre promotes a shift from seeing care as a noun and/or adjective to a verb. We thereby move from a virtue and traits-based system of values to a more interrelational and active one (Held 2006). 'This shift supports [a] mutual and pragmatic recognition of vulnerability, interdependence, and contingency', Jennings et al. (2020) explains, summarising that '[w]hen care is seen as something we actively do—i.e. as a verb—it means that caring is not something we are, but something we do' (p. 193–194).

Nicholson (2005) describes how drama is traditionally associated with the process of identification, where the audience relates to, and empathises with a character. Practitioners such as Brecht (1978) challenged this traditional association, arguing that identification promotes a hierarchical dominance where we simply identify with rather than critically consider presented behaviours. 'He [Brecht] argued that identifying with characters inhibits spectators' ability to contrast the circumstances of their own lives with those portrayed on stage.' (Nicholson 2005: p. 73) This is called an objective distance where rather than seeing the performer as just an actor within the narrative which we may or may not relate to, they are also a person who exists in the real world. The double meaning is that we see the action of the dramatic narrative as more closely linked to our everyday reality. Through self-consciousness and purposeful objective distancing in work like Brecht's, the actor's performance creates a new reality and also reflects elements of our shared reality back to us. More precisely, it consciously reminds us of the reality surrounding the imaginative space of the drama. Here, the audience is posed questions that challenge and disrupt their passivity. This includes a greater awareness that we empathise with those more like us than those we perceive are different. This is a crucial aspect of many approaches to applied drama, where drama is a process and practice through which we might learn and experience something new, and challenge our preconceptions about all manner of things and people, with a focus on active participation over passivity (Nicholson 2005; Prentki and Preston 2008; Hughes and Nicholson 2016).

As Shaughnessy (2015) highlights, empathy has come to be 'used somewhat pejoratively by contemporary performance scholars' (p. 6), however, the concept still influences how applied drama practitioners engage with their participants. Shaughnessy prefers the term 'affective practice', acknowledging the place of kinaesthetic responses, alongside critical understanding in creating 'affect' in applied performance practice. Influential applied theatre scholar Tim Prentki (2023) explores empathy and its role in drama and education following advances in neuroscience which challenge the idea of a Cartesian dualism of mind and body. He argues that 'in the social interactions of our daily lives we are constantly behaving like a theatre audience, reading and responding' (p. 388). He highlights further how theatre actors actions perhaps affect the brains of an audience, whilst a character's actions also potentially affect the brains of the actors' portraying them (p. 389). This points at an intersubjective process of affect, and an intra-subjective one. This focus on 'affect' over effect relates to the work of Thompson (2009). For Thompson, 'attention to affect can be the basis of an ethical focus' which goes beyond the utilitarian 'effect' of applied drama projects (p. 118). Both Shaughnessy and Thompson's conscious move from effect to affect indicate and relate a move from traditional notions of empathy in applied practice. I argue that shifts in theatrical concern as described, including focusing on transitive verbs and affective practice, have signalled a shift from empathy to sympathetic presence in applied drama practice and theory.

Nursing Education, Practice Learning, and Simulation

Moving from the conceptual to the practical, it is worth attending to nursing education in a broader sense. In many countries, nurses must complete practice learning alongside university-based studies to qualify and register as nursing professionals. Broadly speaking, practice learning is learning that takes place in a practice setting rather than a university classroom or skills lab [see: What constitutes Practice-based Learning?|Health Education England (hee.nhs.uk)]. In the UK, this practice is often seen as vital, but it is not entirely uncontentious (Tuckwood et al. 2022). There are worthwhile arguments to be made that though important learning experiences (Cushen-Brewster et al. 2021) the environments and circumstances of these placements are less than conducive to learning. Often students feel these placements solidify a theory-practice gap, and that they are tasked to work as healthcare assistants rather than have the opportunity to learn as part of the healthcare team in the placement (Pearce et al. 2022). Learning in these placements is often contingent on circumstance, guarded by gatekeepers, and unstandardised. The quality of these experiences can vary wildly, and even promote habitual practices that are not evidence-based. Placements are also limited in availability. There is growing evidence that the same or better outcomes are achieved through simulation (Taylor et al. 2021). Moreover, approaches such as healthcare simulation seek to address these issues with practice placements, assuaging the main deficits whilst augmenting the experiences of students in their practice placements. Simulation learning is a wide practice, ranging from demonstrating simple clinical skills to full-blown simulated ward environments, and beyond.

It is reconised that there are 'limitations of clinical placement opportunities [and] restraints on time' in nursing education, so finding new ways to simulate learning is important (Tizzard-Kleister and Jennings 2020: p. 74; Taylor et al. 2021). Reid-Searl et al. (2014) highlight that '[s]imulation learning provides an exciting and relevant solution' in undergraduate nursing education (1202). Although the importance of interpersonal skills and person-centredness has been highlighted as vital for nursing practice (McCormack and McCance 2010, 2016; McCormack et al 2015), these skills prove difficult to teach in SRP (Dingwall et al. 2017; Jennings et al. 2020). Although healthcare simulation has great pedagogical potential as an approach (Aggarwal et al. 2010), Jennings et al. (2020) point towards the need for more 'systematic approaches to training and evaluation in communication skills' (p. 189). This is a well-supported argument in the field (Hallenbeck 2012; Levett-Jones and Lapkin 2014). Doolen et al. (2016) call for improved interpersonal skills in simulation training, whilst highlighting the need for 'stronger simulation designs, standardisation of the process from prebrief to debrief, and faculty training' (301). Siassakos et al. (2011) suggest 'a need for specific training to address such deficiencies in communication [...] such training should start from undergraduate level and continue into postgraduate professional development, involving as many professions as realistically possible' (p. 148).

Healthcare simulation as an approach will be explored more in Chap. 2 and throughout the rest of the book. Broadly, this book argues for a reduction in practice learning placements in favour of increases in simulation learning. Simulation provides a useful stepping stone between conceptual learning and practical applications (Taylor et al. 2021). Furthermore, I argue enhancing simulation learning through drama-based approaches enlivens this process, providing a connecting thread between concepts learned and practices performed. In a specific sense, this study provides evidence that participating in drama-based approaches, with nursing and healthcare as the 'content', should replace some practice learning and traditional simulation hours as it more effectively explores specific key person-centred concepts such as sympathetic presence, and interactive skills more broadly. This is not a call for nurses to take part in any drama. I am certainly not suggesting that taking part in a production of Shakespeare necessarily makes one a better nurse. As mentioned earlier as the central argument of arts in health, taking part in a creative activity like a theatre production may make nurses feel better in general, and perhaps in some specific ways too. I argue drama can do more, and aim to see how drama can enhance nursing education. My argument is for creating and delivering drama-based approaches and processes specifically designed with and for healthcare professionals. A position I hold is that it is not necessarily 'the power' of drama in itself that is helpful, but that the application of particular drama-based approaches has a unique impact on the performance of the person-centred nurse. I am not attempting to directly add to the evidence base for the pursuit of many arts and health research in confirming that taking part in the arts is good for you. Instead, I am more interested in the question of *how* this specific type of art enhances a specific type of healthcare professional education. Pleasingly, without looking for it, this study has significant contributions to both.

It is from this grounding on the shared and divergent concepts of empathy, personhood, sympathetic presence, participation and more that I will dive deeper in Part 1 of this book. Part 1 seeks to produce a shared conceptual frame by surveying the field in Chap. 2, applying Stanislavski's MoPA to nursing education in Chap. 3, and then constructing a shared conceptual frame through an infusion and interweaving of concepts in Chap. 4. Before that, I will present a summary of my doctoral study, the findings from which will take centre stage in Part 2. Part 2 presents four chapters that focus on a discussion of each of the four main themes that were the outcome of my primary research. In these chapters, the findings from my doctoral study will be set in dialogue with the ideas from Part 1.

My Doctoral Study as a Case Study: A Summary

Barring ardent fans of methodological theories of research, or those seeking to replicate a study, the methodology section from a PhD thesis can be dry and uninteresting reading. This summary is given here to provide a fuller picture of my doctoral study,[6] and to align with the main thrust of this book; that specificity is an untapped strength of interdisciplinarity and likewise for the field of arts and health.

The research methodology of my PhD project could be defined as 'applied ethnography'. The primary research of my doctoral study involved the design and delivery of a drama course with participants recruited from the first-year nursing cohort at Ulster University. This process spanned between June 2018 to March 2019. Participants were invited to volunteer to take part in the research, which involved attending a drama-based course designed and co-facilitated by me and contributing research data for the study. Data were collected during these sessions including notes from my participant-observer journal, as well as Creative Personal Reflections (CPR) from the participants. A focus group interview with a sample of participants ($n = 6$) who completed the series of workshops was conducted in March 2019. Once all data had been collected, I thematically analysed the data guided by Gale et al.'s (2013) 'framework method'. This produced four main themes that succinctly represent the findings. These themes are: (1) From self-centredness to person-centredness; (2) Overcoming vulnerability; (3) Attending to others; and (4) Performing presence. The rest of this book will report on the journey I took to arrive at these themes. I will expand on them through discussions involving primary research from my PhD study and a shared conceptual framework developed through research into the field. I will also look ahead at how these themes and the implications of this research might light future paths for the emerging field of drama and

---

[6] One extra thing I wish to mention is that as part of my doctoral study, I engaged in performance practices, self-reflection, and performative auto-ethnography to grapple with the research as well as the question of 'me' as a researcher. Though not a practice-based piece of research, I came to find using my practice as a performer as a natural and invigorating adjunct to my study.

nursing, through the purposefully specific prism of applied drama and person-centred nursing.

What Is Evidence Anyway?

Before moving into Part 1 of the book I wish to present some thoughts on the negotiation between the disciplinary approaches to reviewing literature and the positionality of evidence in each as well as an insight into my position as a researcher approaching this study. One reason to do this is to provide insights into each discipline's approaches, so individuals from one discipline or the other can more easily understand aspects they may be less familiar with from the other discipline. A key topic here is how each discipline has differing points of view of 'evidence'. For instance, in the field of drama strong theoretical conceptualisation can be a more potent identifier of academic rigour and evidence than, say, the design and outcome of an intervention. Many of the seminal examples of research in the field of drama are conceptualisations and theorisations by an individual who is responding to and extending a concept. There is also a strong and growing tradition of performance-based approaches to research which, in broad terms, acknowledges how performing can powerfully conceptualise and articulate aspects of a research project (Mackey 2016). This also means that in the arts journal articles, book chapters, reports, play texts, musical scores, and the like are considered to be weighted equally in terms of what constitutes an idea of 'evidence' in the literature. In contrast, science research has a more defined hierarchy of evidence, and more often uses a structured approach to cultivate evidence. Within the sciences, the strength of a piece of evidence relies more on the ways the researcher follows the scientific method, and how repeatable those results can be for other researchers. Of course, these are generalisations, and many science-based approaches—particularly and increasingly PCN—are quicker to validate different sources of evidence and non-traditional approaches to research, whilst drama research is often conducted through a scientific method.

The disciplines of drama and nursing both acknowledge the split between empirical and conceptual 'evidence'. However, both also acknowledge that this is not binary and should be considered more as a spectrum. The weighting given to empirically and conceptually focused evidence in the two disciplines is often drastically different. For instance, science-based approaches give more weight to recent studies than those published even as recently as 5 years in the past. In the arts, the weight seems to mostly fall from the strength of the concepts explored. What this means for this study in a practical sense is that adopting a singular approach to reviewing from either discipline would invariably cause friction and discomfort with the other. As a result, I have attempted what could be called an 'amorphous' approach. This has involved developing a way forward that speaks to both research languages. For example, I have not shied away from including work published over 5 years ago, though where possible have made efforts to explore and include contemporary publications alongside older ones. Happily, this has meant that seminal but dated texts are presented alongside modern ones. In this way, both old and new co-exist rather than the newer versions replacing older ones.

This section has made it clear there will be elements to this study that are more or less familiar to someone from either field. I discourage a *carte blanché* reading of my work, where all is forgiven in the name of satisfying both disciplines with a 'middle ground'. Instead, this study will borrow from the conceptual idea of metaphorical translation outlined in Tizzard-Kleister and Jennings (2020). Metaphorical translation is an approach where it is acknowledged we cannot fully understand another's perspective, but we can get more adept at metaphorically translating it from our perspective. I have attempted to do this in a broad interdisciplinary sense. This book represents the process and product of a language-learning which serves as a crucial precursor to a translation between the research approaches of drama and nursing as much as it presents a shared conceptual framing between the disciplines that underpin the approach and results of my doctoral study. I see this work as a detailed exploration of how the two fields inter-relate as well as demonstrating one way to undertake the process of interdisciplinary research.

Reflection on My Position as a Researcher and Practitioner

As PCN theorists would say, 'knowing self' is a prerequisite to person-centred practice and research. Meanwhile, drama theorists advocate for self-reflexivity and embed this criticality in their practice and research. As such, I wish to present a critically self-reflective positioning of myself as a researcher and practitioner engaging with this study.

I have been fascinated with the idea of using theatre and performance as an aesthetic framing device through which to explore reality/realities for a long time. In my master's studies I explored how contemporary participatory performance described by authors like Claire Bishop (2012) in many ways discourages a co-construction of this frame between audience and spectator. I explored how many contemporary artists framed their work as involving meaningful participation, but in reality, gave audiences little autonomy to change the aesthetic frame of the work. As a result, the audience's freedom to act was bound by the parameters of the work put in place by the artist, in turn limiting the scope of the aesthetic frame. I consider that this reflects a broader social and philosophical position in the arts, particularly in its role within the 'entertainment economy', drawing on Adorno's notions of cultural economics shaping political and social normativity (Adorno 2016). In this context, my work explored how in many examples of contemporary participatory theatre the autonomy afforded the participants was deeply linked to neoliberal political concerns (Kester 2012; Boucher 2013), reflecting a limited scope for people to take autonomous action in their real lives. Simply, I assert that projects such as those described by Bishop (2012) present an image of participation, not true autonomy. This led me to further questions about the potential of performance art as a meaningful participatory experience, and how creativity is often seen as a liberator but can be constricting.

I sought to address this in my practical work. To do so I developed several short participatory pieces in which the actions of participants were explicitly counteracted, heightened, or given 'complete' creative freedom. I sought to highlight both this false autonomy in similar performance practice and everyday life. For example, in my short one-to-one performance *It's just a game* I invited members of the public to join me for an endgame of chess.[7] The set-up of the performance was minimal, and instructions were infrequent and purposefully vague. After a few turns, I began to cheat. The participants' responses to this 'breaking of the frame'—both that of chess as a game and the frame of the performance—are the central premise of the performance. This cheating escalated until I inevitably won. At the time, I likened the loss of autonomy for the participant to the general loss of autonomy experienced by many in the UK and further afield due to neoliberal ideology stultifying free-thinking and genuine creative self-expression.

A central argument I have developed in response to the reception to, and my experience with, the above example is the importance for artists to allow participants to reshape, and meaningfully affect, the work they participated in. My results showed how when we do so, we can come together and use theatre as a safe pedagogical and dialogic space to challenge stereotypical representations. But often the first step lay in tearing away the facade of the aesthetic frame and challenging our shared conception of what it means to be a performer and what the role of a spectator is. I discovered that exploring participation in theatre in this way creates a powerful place in which we might reshape our histories and futures. In the case of *It's just a game* (which developed into a larger scale, group participative game of 'human chess') by breaking the frame of the game, I invite the audience to choose how they wish to reconstruct it. The inevitability of my winning, I realised, was an unconscious reference to the fallacy of the artist who never relinquishes 'control' of their aesthetic framework, a sentiment I soon came to see as something I struggle with creatively.

My work has attempted to theoretically and practically position the use of participative performance as a framing through which aesthetics, identities, and meaning might emerge. This is similar to how Norman (2012, 2015) suggests theatre may be used almost as a 'scientific instrument' with which we can explore emergent phenomena. My work extended to include how this has the potential to move beyond mimetic representation as a form of identity construction to instead construct a broader range of identities through Hallward's (2006) reading of Deleuzian theories. In short, exploring how we can perform different roles and identities in these performances that solidify or challenge our identities in real life. Through experimenting in a theatrical frame, we discover the potential to perform in everyday life. In this way, participative performance would be a place and practice through which

---

[7] An 'endgame' is the late stages of the game of chess, where only a few different pieces remain for either side. Some people purposefully set up different endgame situations with a variety of remaining pieces and in different positions to practice how to navigate them. Endgames are often presented as a problem to solve.

we might discover and develop a deeper 'knowing self', as I would soon find is a key piece in the PCNF.

It has been an eventful journey developing this position from the beginning of my doctorate in 2018, to the development of this book summarising it. Though I still consider the above position broadly representative of my current one, I have had to reconsider some aspects. A key point I have had to confront is the shift in perspective from the contemporary participatory performances explored by Bishop (2012) to the community-based approaches of applied drama, such as those explored by Thompson (2009, 2015) amongst many others. I am happy to admit that at the time the term 'applied theatre', and the insightful work completed over some six decades or more was unfamiliar to me as I began my doctorate. Discovering this field was, for me, a paradigm shift. One of the most prolific applied drama practitioners and theorists in the last two decades James Thompson (2015) critiques both the perspective of projects analysed by Bishop (2012) and Bishop's critique and positioning of participatory art. Thompson explains that these contemporary practices rely on shock, disturbance, and disruption in that they do not account for the desires of the attending audience. This leaves the desires and perspectives of the audience under-explored and a mystery to the artist. Thompson is therefore critical of Bishop's central arguments on the emancipatory potential within these more professionally-based, contemporary works. Instead, he points towards the long history of applied drama, particularly how applied drama often involves working meaningfully[8] with many different participants in a broad range of contexts. Though I am less critical of projects explored by Bishop, I wholeheartedly agree with Thompson's critique of artists unconcerned with their audience's desires as this too easily falls into what Harvie (2013) has called 'prosumerism'. This is where a participant both produces and consumes aesthetic content with little meaning beyond entertainment, cheap shocks, and a semi-interesting topic of discussion with friends and family.

In recent hindsight, I hope to experiment with *It's Just a Game* in future, undercut the inevitability of my control and find a way to directly ask my participant a simple question towards the end of the performance—'how do you want this game to end?' I see this as promoting a new starting point for building a framework together. Nicholson (2017) highlights how participant agency is 'illusory' in many examples of prosumer-style participatory performance which manipulates and commodifies the 'affective labour' of the participant, arguing the need to 'revitalise the conventional role of the artist as social critic' (p.117, p. 110). As a result, how both the artist and the audience co-construct the frame through which the performance is perceived needs to be reconsidered to ensure the participant has the opportunity to make meaningful additions to the fabric of the performance. What this relationship

---

[8] A loaded term I am very purposefully using here. In this case, its use is to point to the notion of value and meaning in applied theatre work. This is an area of seemingly ingrained debate in the field, and one that I suspect serves to define the field more than most wish to admit. For me, it is the search for meaning and value in applied drama work that often leads to and provides its very meaning. I argue this facet sets applied drama apart from its 'non-applied' counterparts, which may be more content to not explore that very question.

relies on, I have come to realise, is care. In my studies, I have been influenced by the Ethics of Care (Held 2006), and Thompson's (2015, 2023) Aesthetics of Care, both of which I have already briefly mentioned, and I will explore in more detail later in this book. The practice of creating caring relationships in a performance hopefully translates neatly to doing so in real life. Another significant shift for me has been in moving to a practice of facilitation (Preston 2016) through an applied drama tradition rather than as an 'artist'. However, Hepplewhite (2020) reminds us the term artist certainly applies to applied theatre practitioners. What this resonates with is the role of the person-centred nurse shifting from a person who simply delivers care transactionally, to one that facilitates person-centred care (Lieshout and Cardiff 2015).

Shaughnessy (2015) suggests an approach of participant-centred pedagogy as important for applied drama, where an atmosphere is created but not defined by the bodies in space and where 'the perceiving subject is in a state of becoming through the process of being transported in an affective and affecting event' (p. 210). If the aesthetic frame offered by the artist aims towards a conscious social critique, this frame should always be made complete in conjunction with the participant—Shaughnessy's 'perceiving subject'. It must meanwhile incorporate a participant-centred approach to work together in a process towards the mutual creation of this critique through an 'affecting event'. I add that this event inherently involves a caring relationship, whether the experience is 'caring' or not. Simply, applied drama should strive to bring people together, to explore themselves and what is important to them, in an active process and through an engaging event—and where the people involved are in a caring relationship. Similarly, the 'frame' presented by the person-centred nurse when engaging with others is only complete with the contribution of others. Whilst developing the conceptual frame and reviewing literature for this study, Goffman's (1990) dramaturgy of everyday life and returning to Stanislavski's (1990) Method of Physical Action offered a compelling starting point into which to approach thinking as 'the artist' providing such a dramaturgical frame.

Through attending to key concepts, presenting my doctoral study as a case study, exploring distinctions of how each field views evidence, and positioning myself within the study, this chapter has laid the ground for Part 1 of this book. Part 1 will explore and present a shared conceptual frame for working across applied drama and person-centred nursing, beginning with Chap. 2 which reviews the field to explore the intersections of drama and nursing.

References

Adorno T. (trans. Redmond D. http://members.efn.org/~dredmond/ndtrans.html, accessed May 2016) Negative Dialectics

Aggarwal R, Mytton OT, Derbrew M, Hananel D, Heydenburg M, Issenberg B, MacAulay C, Mancini ME, Morimoto T, Soper N, Ziv A, Reznick R (2010) Training and simulation for patient safety. BMJ Qual Saf:34–43

APPG (2017) Creative health: the arts for health and wellbeing. All-Party Parliamentary Group, London

Arveklev S, Wigert H, Berg L, Lepp M (2020) Specialist nursing students' experiences of learning through drama in paediatric care. Nurse Educ Pract 43:1–6

Baxter V, Low KE (2017) Performing health and wellbeing. Bloomsbury Methuen Drama, London

Bishop C (2012) Artificial Hells. Verso, London

Bloom P (2018) Against empathy: the case for rational compassion. Vintage, London

Boal A (1998) Theatre of the oppressed. Pluto Press, London

Boucher G (2013) Adorno: reframed, I.B. Tauris, London

Brecht B (1978) Brecht on theatre. Methuen, London

Brodzinski E (2010) Theatre in health and care. Palgrave, Basingstoke

Brodzinski E (2014) Performance anxiety the relationship between social and aesthetic drama in medicine and health. In: Bates V, Bleakley A, Goodman S (eds) Medicine, health and the arts: approaches to the medical humanities. Routledge, Abingdon, pp 165–185

Clift S, Camic P (eds) (2016) Creative arts, health, and wellbeing: international perspectives on practice, policy, and research. Oxford University Press, Oxford

Cunico L, Sartori R, Marognolli O, Meneghini A (2012) Developing empathy in nursing students: a cohort longitudinal study. J Clin Nurs 21(13–14):2016–2025

Cushen-Brewster N, Barker A, Driscoll-Evans P, Wigens L, Langton H (2021) The experiences of adult nursing students completing a placement during the COVID-19 pandemic. Br J Nurs 30:21

Damsgaard J (2020) Integrating the arts and humanities into nursing. Nurs Philos 22:2

Dewing J, Eide T, McCormack B (2017) Philosophical perspectives on person-centredness for healthcare research. In: McCormack B, Dulmen S, Eide H, Skovdahl K, Eide T (eds) Person-Centred nursing research. Wiley Blackwell, Chichester, pp 19–30

Dewing J, McCormack B, McCance T (eds) (2021) Person-Centred nursing research: methodology, methods and outcomes. Springer, London

Dingwall L, Fenton J, Kelly TB, Lee J (2017) Sliding doors: did drama-based inter-professional education improve the tensions round person-centred nursing and social care delivery for people with dementia: a mixed method exploratory study. Nurse Educ Today 51:1–7

Doolen J, Mariani B, Atz T, Horsley TL, Rourke JO, McAfee K, Cross CL (2016) High-fidelity simulation in undergraduate nursing education: a review of simulation reviews. Clin Simul Nurs 12(7):290–302

Ekebergh M, Lepp M, Dahlberg K (2004) Reflective learning with Drama in Nursing Education—a Swedish attempt to overcome the theory praxis gap. Nurse Educ Today 24:622–628

Fancourt D (2017) Arts in health: designing and researching interventions. Oxford University Press, Oxford

Fancourt D, Finn S (2019) What is the evidence on the role of the arts in improving health and well-being? WHO, Helsinki

Fancourt D, Warran K, Aughterson H (2020) Evidence summary for policy: the role of arts in improving health & wellbeing, Report to the Department for Digital, Culture, Media, & Sport

Gale N, Heath G, Cameron E, Rashid S, Redwood S (2013) Using the framework method for the analysis of qualitative data in multi-disciplinary health research. BMC Med Res Methodol 13:117. 09/02/2018 [Online] Available from: https://bmcmedresmethodol.biomedcentral.com/articles/10.1186/1471-2288-13-117

Gilligan C (1990) In a different voice: psychological theory and women's development. Harvard University Press, Cambridge, MA

Goffman E (1990) The presentation of self in everyday life. Penguin, London

Hallenbeck VJ (2012) Use of high-fidelity simulation for staff education/development: a systematic review of the literature. J Nurses Staff Dev 28(6):260–269

Hallward P (2006) Out of this world. Verso, London

Harvie J (2013) Fair play: performance and neoliberalism. Palgrave Macmillan, London

Heggestad AKT, Nortvedt P, Christiansen B, Konow-Lund A (2016) Undergraduate nursing students' ability to empathize: a qualitative study. Nurs Ethics 25(6):786–795

Held V (2006) The ethics of care: personal, political, and global. Oxford University Press, Oxford

Hepplewhite K (2020) The applied theatre artist: responsivity and expertise in practice. Palgrave Macmillan, London

Hochschild AR (1983) The managed heart. University of California Press, Berkeley

Hoffman ML (2000) Empathy and moral development: implications for caring and justice. Cambridge University Press, Cambridge

Hojat M (2009) Empathy in patient care: antecedents, development, measurement, and outcomes. Springer, New York

Hughes J, Nicholson H (eds) (2016) Critical perspectives on applied theatre. Cambridge University Press, Cambridge

Jacobs G (2015) The Currentness of person-Centred practice. Int Pract Dev J 5

Jacobs G, Lieshout F, Borg M, Ness O (2017) Being a person-centred researcher: principles and methods for doing research in a person-centred way. In: McCormack B, Dulmen S, Eide H, Skovdahl K, Eide T (eds) Person-Centred healthcare research. Wiley Blackwell, Chichester, pp 51–60

Jeffrey D (2017) Communicating with a human voice: developing a relational model of empathy. J R Coll Physicians Edinb 47(3):266–270

Jennings M, Deeny P, Tizzard-Kleister K (2020) Acts of care: applied drama, 'sympathetic presence' and person-centred nursing. In: Stuart Fisher A, Thompson J (eds) Performing care: new perspectives on socially engaged performance. Manchester University Press, Manchester, pp 187–203

Kester G (2012) The noisy optimism of immediate action: theory, practice, and pedagogy in contemporary art. Art J 71(2):86–99

Kirk TW (2007) Beyond empathy: clinical intimacy in nursing practice. Nurs Philos 8:233–243

Kitwood T (1997) Dementia reconsidered: the person comes first. Open University Press, Buckingham

Klimecky O, Leiberg S, Ricard M, Singer T (2014) Differential pattern of functional brain plasticity after compassion and empathy training. Soc Cogn Affect Neurosci 9(6):873–879

Kyle R, Bastow F, Harper-McDonald B, Jeram T, Zahid Z, Nizamuddin M, Mahoney C (2023) Effects of student-led drama on nursing students' attitudes to interprofessional working and nursing advocacy: a pre-test post-test educational intervention study. Nurse Educ Today 123:1–11

Levett-Jones T, Lapkin S (2014) A systematic review of the effectiveness of simulation debriefing in health professional education. Nurse Educ Today 34:58–63

Lieshout F, Cardiff S (2015) Reflections on being and becoming a person-centred facilitator. Int Pract Dev J 5. Available from: https://www.fons.org/library/journal/volume5-person-centredness-suppl/article4. Accessed 09-03-2018]

Mackey S (2016) Applied theatre and practice as research: polyphonic conversations. Res Drama Educ : The Journal of Applied Theatre and Performance 21(4):478–491

McCance T, McCormack B, Tizzard-Kleister K, Wallace L (2021) Being sympathetically presence. In: McCormack B, McCance T, Bulley C, McMillan A, Martin S, Brown D (eds) Fundamentals of person-centred healthcare practice. Wiley-Blackwell, Chichester

McCormack B, McCance T (2006) Development of a framework for person-centred nursing. J Adv Nurs 56(5):472–479

McCormack B, McCance T (2010) Person-centred nursing: theory and practice. Wiley-Blackwell, Chichester

McCormack B, Borg M, Cardiff S, Dewing J, Jacobs G, Janes N, Karlsson B, McCance T, Mekki T, Propock D, van Lieshout F, Wilson V (2015) Person-Centredness - the 'state' of the art, in International Practice Development Journal, 5(1)

McCormack B, McCance T (eds) (2016) Person-centred practice in nursing and health care, 2nd edn. Wiley-Blackwell, Chichester

McCormack B, McCance T, Bulley C, McMillan A, Martin S, Brown D (eds) (2021) Fundamentals of person-centred healthcare practice. Wiley-Blackwell, Chichester

Mearns D, Thorne B (2007) Person-centred counselling in action. Sage Publications, London

Mermikides A (2020) Performance, medicine and the human. Methuen Drama, London

Mohammad E, Onavbavba G, Wilson D, Adigwe O (2022) Understanding the nature and sources of conflict among healthcare professionals in Nigeria: a qualitative study. J Multidiscip Healthc 15:1979–1995

Neelands J, Belfiore E, Firth C, Hart N, Perrin L, Holdaway D, Woddis J (2015) Enriching Britain: culture, creativity and growth. The Warwick Commission

Nicholson H (2005) Applied Drama: the gift of theatre. Palgrave Macmillan, London

Nicholson H (2017) Affective Labours of cultural participation. In: Harpin A, Nicholson H (eds) Performance and participation: practices, audiences, politics. Palgrave Macmillan, London, pp 105–127

Nnate D, Nashwan A (2023) Emotional intelligence and delivering bad news in professional nursing practice. Cereus 15:6

Noddings N (2013) Freire, Buber, and care ethics on dialogue in teaching. In: Lake R, Kress T, Giroux H, Aronowitz S, Freire P, McLaren P (eds) Paulo Freire's intellectual roots: towards historicity in praxis. Bloomsbury, London, pp 89–100

Noonan I, Rafferty AM, Browne J (2016) Creative arts in health professional education and practice: a case study reflection and evaluation of a complex intervention to deliver the Culture and Care programme at the Florence Nightingale School of Nursing and Midwifery, King's College London. In: Clift S, Camic P (eds) Creative arts, health, and wellbeing: International perspectives on practice, policy, and research. Oxford University Press, Oxford, pp 309–316

Norman SJ (2012) Theatre as an art of emergence and individuation. Archit Theory Rev 17(1):117–133

Norman SJ (2015) Theater and ALife art: modeling open and closed systems. Artif Life 21(3):344–353

Nunes P, Williams S, Sa B, Stevenson K (2011) A study of empathy decline in students from five health disciplines during their first year of training. Int J Med Educ 2:12–17

Nursing and Midwifery Council (NMC) (2015) The code for nurses and midwives. NMC, London. Available from: https://www.nmc.org.uk/globalassets/sitedocuments/nmc-publications/nmc-code.pdf. Accessed 30 Oct 2018

Nursing and Midwifery Council (NMC) (2018) Future nurse: standards for proficiency and practice for registered nurses. NMC. Available from: future-nurse-proficiencies.pdf (nmc.org.uk). Accessed 1 June 2021

Pearce R, Topping A, Willis C (2022) Enhancing healthcare students' clinical placement experiences. In: Nursing Standard. RCNI

Prentki T (2023) A short essay on empathy, drama, and a new curriculum. Res Drama Educ 28(3):387–391

Prentki T, Preston S (eds) (2008) The applied theatre reader. Routledge, London

Preston S (2016) Applied theatre: facilitation: pedagogies, practices, resistance. Bloomsbury Methuen, London

Readman G (2023) National drama's response to the arts in schools review. National Drama. (National Drama's Response to the Arts in Schools Review—NATIONAL DRAMA)

Reid-Searl K, Mcallister M, Dwyer T, Krebs K, Anderson C, Quinney L, McLellan S (2014) Little people, big lessons: an innovative strategy to develop interpersonal skills in undergraduate nursing students. Nurse Educ Today 34:1201–1206

Rogers C (1961) On becoming a person, a therapist's view of psychotherapy. Houghton-Mifflin, Boston

Shaughnessy N (2015) Applying performance: live art, socially engaged theatre and affective practice. Palgrave Macmillan, London

Siassakos D et al (2011) Team communication with patient actors: findings from a multisite simulation study. Simul Healthc 6(3):143–149

Smith P (1992) The emotional labour of nursing: its impact on interpersonal relations, management and educational environments. Palgrave, Basingstoke

Smith K (2016) Reflection and person-centredness in practice development. Int Pract Dev J 6:1

Stanislavski C (1990) An actor's handbook. Methuen, London

Storaker A, Nåden D, Sæteren B (2017) From painful busyness to emotional immunization: nurses' experiences of ethical challenges. Nurs Ethics 24(5):556–568

Stuart Fisher A, Thompson J (eds) (2020) Performing care: new perspectives on socially engaged performance. Manchester University Press, Manchester

Taylor N, Wyres M, Green A, Hennessy-Priest K, Phillips C, Daymond E, Love R, Johnson R, Wright J (2021) Developing and piloting a simulated placement experience for students. Br J Nurs 30:13

Thompson J (2009) Performance affects: applied theatre and the end of effect. Palgrave Macmillan, Basingstoke

Thompson J (2015) Towards an aesthetics of care. Res Drama Educ. The Journal of Applied Theatre and Performance 20(4):430–441

Thompson J (2023) Care aesthetics: for artful care and careful art. Routledge, London

Tizzard-Kleister K, Jennings M (2020) "Breath, belief, focus, touch": applied puppetry in simulated role play for person-Centred nursing education. Appl Theatre Res 8(1):73–87

Tronto J (2013) Caring democracy: markets, equality, and justice. New York University Press, New York

Tuckwood S, Carey L, O'Gorman J (2022) It's broken, let's fix it—the future of UK nurse undergraduate education. J Clin Nurs 31(15–16):20–22

Vickhoff B (2023) Why art? The role of arts in art and health. Front Psychol 14

Ward J, Cody J, Schaal M, Hojat M (2012) The empathy enigma: an empirical study of decline in empathy among undergraduate nursing students. J Prof Nurs 28(1):34–40

Wasylko Y, Stickley T (2003) Theatre and pedagogy: using drama in mental health nurse education. Nurse Educ Today 23:443–448

White M (2009) Arts development in community health: a social tonic. Radcliffe, Oxford

Williams J, Stickley T (2010) Empathy and nurse education. Nurse Educ Today 30(8):752–755

Yakhforoshha A, Emami SAH, Mohammadi N, Cheraghi M, Mojtahedzadeh R, Mahmoodi-Bakhtiari B, Shirazi M (2017) Developing an integrated educational simulation model by considering art approach: teaching empathetic communication skills. Eur J Pers Cent Healthc 5(1):154–165

Part I

Conceptualising Applied Drama and Person-centred Nursing

Exploring the Terrain of Drama and Nursing

Developing Person-Centred Healthcare Practices: The Key Challenges

There is a growing interest for care as an experience, characterised by the interpersonal skill of the practitioner delivering it. The 1993 General Medical Council (GMC) report *Tomorrow's Doctors* was influential in creating a shift in a collective mindset in health education from just imparting knowledge to students to developing a robust ability for critical analysis. This also began the move towards highlighting features of the work of healthcare staff such as communication as skills, rather than just inherent traits and values (GMC 1993). As mentioned in Chap. 1, this focus has only sharpened as seen in the NMC (2018) code which gives communication an entire appendix. This being said, there are still enduring inconsistencies in how communication is taught (Randle et al. 2003; Williams and Stickley 2010; Lawrence and Wier 2018). After the publication of *The Francis Report* (Francis 2013), a report into the drastic shortcomings of specific healthcare environments in Mid-Staffordshire, how healthcare staff might better engage with patients was summarised as 'the 6 C's' by the NHS. These six C's are 'Care', 'Compassion', 'Competence', 'Communication', 'Courage', and 'Commitment'. Lawrence and Wier (2018) highlight the difficulty of teaching newly required value sets, such as the 6 C's, where though students might be able to 'recite the 6 Cs, few of them had a practical working knowledge of how these might be applied in practice' (p. 59).

The National Archives (TNA) produced a report on complaints across the NHS, pinpointing 'many accounts of patients not being treated with dignity or respect' (The National Archives (TNA) 2013: p. 16). Requirements for all healthcare students have grown to include a respect for patients in a more holistic sense. Paraphrasing Willson (2006), students and staff must begin to think ethically and morally about the care they give. Jennings et al. (2020) show how complaints from patients in the NHS are often about communication issues, and how these issues are perhaps ironically best resolved by reestablishing effective communication. They

© The Author(s), under exclusive license to Springer Nature Switzerland AG 2024

K. Tizzard-Kleister, *Applied Drama and Person-Centred Nursing*, https://doi.org/10.1007/978-3-031-77208-5_2

highlight how in the Patient Client Council (PCC) 2016–17 annual report, 'communication problems and staff attitude [are] the basis for 28.5 per cent of total complaints [whilst] the same report shows that the most effective methods for resolving complaints, all of which depend on interpersonal communication, account for 82.5 percent of all resolutions' (Jennings et al. 2020: p. 187). Emma Brodzinski (2014) highlights similar findings by exploring the work of Bleakley et al. (2011), who found 70% of observed medical errors were due to poor communication. Brodzinski concludes that around half of the resolutions to these errors were achieved through 'better education in communication and teamwork' (2014: p. 183). This evidence suggests that improved communication skills could resolve many of the issues faced within the NHS—and health care globally. Yet these so-called soft skills are often neglected within medical and nursing training in favour of a focus on technical or 'hard skills' (Monden et al. 2016).

Another under-considered area in nursing education is a robust explanation of the emotional work of a nurse and how negotiating one's emotions affects communication (Schlegel et al. 2014: p. 666). This includes a recognised lack of emotional support for nursing students throughout their studies, practice learning placements, and transition to work (Williams and Stickley 2010). Moreover, little of the nursing curriculum is given over to helping students understand the emotional demands of nursing work including how to avoid emotional indifference (Heggestad et al. 2016). As a result, how this might affect the practitioner's body language and ability to communicate is also under-considered (Yakhforoshha et al. 2017). For Leahy (2002) '[t]he first step' to working with difficult emotions 'involves attending to the emotion' rather than ignoring or suppressing them (p. 180). Paying conscious attention to emotions is therefore 'related to less anxiety and less depression' (Ibid: p. 187).

Both the lack of focus given to emotional engagement and the difficulty in finding time to attend to emotions could be a contributor to a global shortfall in healthcare staff. Retention is a key issue for healthcare. Wilson et al. (2015) identify four factors that when enhanced improve care as well as retention: working environment, social support, less stress and burnout, and satisfaction with work (p. 91). Approaches such as PCN are well suited to addressing this. PCN holistically and respectfully views all persons in healthcare as unique and reassesses the primacy of 'hard' skills over 'soft' skills, in 'a collaborative process between the person seeking help and the practitioner in various contexts' (Hummelvoll et al. 2015: p. 4). PCN is a nursing approach based on putting the concept of personhood and the quality of person-to-person contact at the centre of nursing (Kitwood 1997; McCormack and McCance 2010, 2016). In doing so, PCN highlights the importance of building relationships and interpersonal skills as vital for shifting from frequently uncompassionate 'mechanistic care' (de Zulueta 2013) to what McCormack and McCance term 'affective care' (2010: p. 25). PCN researchers advocate for care environments which promote innovation and risk-taking to facilitate this (Ibid: 78–83). Some have called for 'the use of educational interventions that explicitly facilitate emotional development and enable students to develop their own innate empathic capacity and self-awareness' (Williams and Stickley 2010: p. 755). The arts have been a major area of collaboration to this effect (Perry et al. 2011; Brodzinski 2010, 2014; Fancourt 2017), not least in healthcare simulation. However, even with the support of arts-based approaches, there are still significant challenges to face in moving towards person-centredness in healthcare.

One potential root cause of the many issues that face healthcare in becoming person-centred is the predominance of the biomedical model of care. Fancourt (2017) describes how 'Germ Theory' created a shift in how the Western world viewed health. Now humanity had a provable, material, and measurable culprit of ill health; the microbial 'germ', giving rise to 'the biomedical model' of health (Ibid, p. 23). With a deeper understanding of bacteria, 'health was seen as an absence of disease measured by empirical markers' and 'the medical practitioner became the privileged interpreter of illness' (Brodzinski 2010: p. 4, p. 31). Through the calamity of the First World War and into the height of the Modernist period healthcare settings were further sanitised and controlled, with things like art, practitioner–patient relationships and spirituality seen as wasteful and unnecessary (Fancourt 2017; Mermikides 2020).

Brodzinski (2014) points to Foucault as a key cultural and philosophical influence on the development of biomedical notions of health. For Brodzinski, it was Foucault's focus on power that highlighted how 'the person in authority (the doctor) actualizes disease' (p. 169) and creates a diagnostic gaze where the sole defender of the risks, dangers, and harms of ill health is the medical professional. As Alice O'Grady (2017) illustrates, the cultural perception of risk as a concept throughout the Modernist period was as the probability of danger, but in more recent times, risk has come to be perceived as synonymous with danger, and therefore no longer something to be mitigated against but to be avoided entirely (p. 6). We can see how this resulted in the work of healthcare staff focusing on harm and illness prevention by not just reducing dangerous and uncertain risks but guarding against *any* form of risk, for example, through adopting systems to avoid instances like operating on the wrong leg, in-hospital injury, patient mismanagement, and so on. As a result, in secure and sterile care environments deviation from crucial systems and protocols is automatically considered risky. Although the positive effects of the biomedical model cannot be denied, and risk management approaches have emerged and succeeded in avoiding certain dangerous risks, focusing on finding and solving problems may 'overlook individuals and their needs' (Brodzinski 2010: p. 18).

Solely developing technical competence 'loses sight of the patient' (Williams and Stickley 2010: p. 754) by neglecting the importance of interpersonal relationships, and the skills required to develop them as well as the place of these skills and relationships in mitigating against emotional harm. As Buxton (2011) highlights, '[t]o become effective, empathetic practitioners, students need to overcome their anxiety and fear' (p. 31). Moreover, without the value systems often described as fundamental to nursing 'there is a risk that nursing is performed as tasks or actions with no deeper meaning' (Arveklev et al. 2015: p. 12). PCN aims to move towards a holistic and values-based consideration of nursing. It is an approach that privileges the personhood of all people involved in a care process, advocating for creating and sustaining positive working cultures and staff-patient relationships (McCormack

2001a, b; McCance 2003; McCormack and McCance 2010). As Dingwall et al. (2017) make clear even with innovative and effective methods showing potential to develop these skills in students, there is still a pervasive and prevailing risk aversion that halts growth.

Brodzinski suggests the 'care sector can be seen as having a risk-averse culture' (2010: p. 18), which drama-based approaches can help to address, specifically through enhancing healthcare simulation. McCormack and McCance (2010) criticise this risk aversion as leading to a 'task-based' form of care in nursing (p. 101). This task-based approach creates healthcare practitioners who Ritzer (2004) would call 'McDoctors'—or in our case 'McNurses'[1]—'who deal with minor healthcare problems in the quickest/most cost-effective manner, thus limiting the quality of patient contact' (Goodwin and Deady 2013: p. 126). Brodzinski's later work (2014) goes further and positions 'an emphasis on success within health settings' as a contributing factor to sustaining 'a culture of risk aversion' (p. 182). How risk, and more precisely risk aversion, affect nursing and influence how drama and the arts can be applied to the profession is explored more in Chap. 4, where a conjoined conceptual frame is discussed.

Person-Centred Nursing, the Antidote?

It can be said that a key goal of PCN is to be an antidote to the proliferation of risk-averse 'McNurses', specifically by highlighting nursing-specific metrics of success as equally important to medicine-specific metrics. Agreeing with Brodzinski, I argue that drama-based approaches offer the perfect environments and effective methods to enhance and administer this antidote. PCN privileges the personhood of all people involved in a care process, advocating for creating and sustaining positive working cultures and staff-patient relationships (McCormack 2001a, b; McCance 2003; McCormack and McCance 2010). It can be said that PCN is an attempt to personalise healthcare, addressing, amongst other concerns, poor communication in healthcare settings (McCormack et al. 2015; Belfast Health and Social Care Trust 2017; Patient Client Council 2017). Whereas PCN continues to be adopted globally, research has mostly explored the notion of care and what makes care person-centred. A recognised deficit is research into how PCN can change cultures and sustain those changes to promote positive person-to-person relationships (McCormack et al. 2015).[2]

---

[1] I reject the outright criticism of people who work for large organisations, such as McDonald's. The criticism I intend is to the systems perpetuated by large corporations that de-centralise people in their operations, leading to workers who are seen as, and often feel like, just cogs in a machine.

[2] This has developed into work on what makes curricula (as a systems approach, and not just one-off curriculum events like a single module) person-centred. This has led to the development of the Person-Centred Curriculum Framework (Cook et al. 2022) published after the conclusion of my doctoral study, and certainly, a relevant point of comparison and often convergence to the features of the drama course developed as part of my doctoral research.

Jennings et al. (2020) explain how PCN 'hinges on the primary concept of 'personhood', whereby an individual is treated as a person with their characteristics, values, beliefs, attitudes, unique life story, and future goals' (p. 192). Personhood, as McCormack & McCance define it, plays a central role in PCN. Broadly, personhood is articulated through a sense of self and the relationship between the self and other elements of 'being' including authenticity, morality, reflectivity, and the embodiment of these elements (McCormack and McCance 2010). Some practitioners have crafted transposable frameworks to guide practitioners in a variety of healthcare settings. One such framework is the PCNF (McCormack and McCance 2010; Dewing et al. 2021). The framework has been carefully developed since its inception, expanding in scope to encompass how to incite and sustain cultural changes in healthcare environments ((McCormack and McCance 2006, 2010, 2016). Moreover, in the second edition of their seminal text McCormack and McCance expanded the PCNF to the PCPF, reflecting the utility of the framework beyond nursing and into other areas of healthcare such as social work, healthcare assistance, and so on. As this study focuses on nursing, the PCNF will be more readily drawn from than the PCPF (for the PCNF see Fig. 2.1 overleaf).

The PCNF has been adopted in a variety of areas and institutes across the globe, including the UK, Canada, Australia, Scandinavia, and more (McCormack et al. 2015). Most importantly for the context of the case study of my doctoral study, the PCNF has underpinned the Nursing degree curriculum at Ulster University since 2014. This underpinning has attempted to guide students and professionals in the creation and continuation of cultures and attitudes that actively enable engagement with care practices where 'the relationship between the nurses and the person being cared for is paramount' (McCormack and McCance 2010: p. 27). As it is, the framework addresses 'person-centredness' throughout the whole system of care and nursing as a totality. It does so by considering multiple levels of healthcare. This began in the early versions with macro elements including features such as 'health and social care policy', 'workforce developments', and so on. In general, this section of the framework looks at how nursing and healthcare can encompass person-centredness, and promote person-centred culture in the broadest terms. This addresses how—arguably—nursing theory has disproportionately focused on the caring exchange and less so on how nursing concepts can affect healthcare policy and culture more widely. As you will notice above, in the most recent version of the PCNF (Dewing et al. 2021), these were replaced with the 'metaparadigm of nursing' (Hardy 1978). The change still captures the notion of a 'macrocontext' for person-centred nursing, whilst highlighting the nursing-specific paradigms of that wider context.

Drilling down from here the framework looks at the prerequisites for one to be a person-centred nurse. For instance, being 'professionally competent' or showing 'commitment to the job'. This is preceded by a description of what makes a PCN care environment. This comprises 'effective staff relationships', 'supportive organisational systems', 'potential for innovation and risk-taking', and more. From here specific processes are outlined, like 'being sympathetically present' or 'providing holistic care'. Optimistically, the framework is intended as a guiding system 'rather

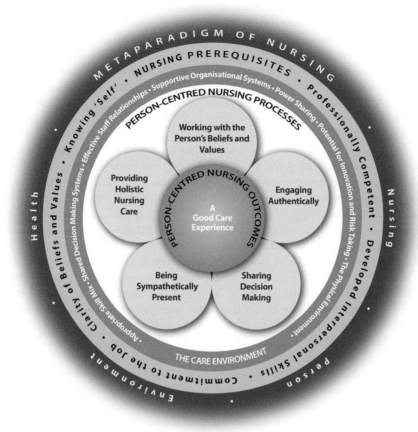

Fig. 2.1 The Person-Centred Nursing Framework, Dewing et al. 2021. With permission from: McCormack, B., McCance, T. (2021). The Person-Centred Nursing Framework. In: Dewing, J., McCormack, B., McCance, T. (eds) Person-centred Nursing Research: Methodology, Methods and Outcomes. Springer, Cham, Springer Nature. https://doi.org/10.1007/978-3-030-27868-7_2

than […] yet another technical approach to measuring outcomes' (Wilson and McCance 2015: p. 8). Whilst the framework 'sets out the elements and processes that lead to person-centred nursing' (Niessen and Jacobs 2015: p. 1), this is not designed as a tick-box exercise and instead presents a deeper challenge to those who wish to actively approach PCN and meaningfully reflect on their assumptions, personhood, and positions as they relate to PCN. This being said, whilst the framework articulates what it means to be person-centred it is recognised that in practice, 'less is known about whether education aimed at person-centred care can prepare students for it and, if so, how' (Ibid). One area that this research study seeks to develop more knowledge in is the process of 'sympathetic presence'. Chapter 1 presented a definition of the term by drawing across the disciplines of drama and nursing, highlighting the resonance of the term, and the potential for it to serve as the lynchpin in this interdisciplinary study. A central premise of this study is the unique ways in which arts, specifically drama, enhance the understanding and practice of sympathetic presence. To outline why, it is necessary to outline how arts and drama have been applied to health and healthcare more broadly.

Arts and Health

'Arts and Health' is a field interested in exploring the cross over between the arts and health in a variety of areas and has seen tremendous growth in the last two decades (White 2009; Baxter and Low 2017; Fancourt 2017). In a general sense, art interventions in healthcare have helped to co-construct a 'new language with which to discuss health, often empowering patients to feel visible at a time when their sense of identity is fragile' (Willson 2006: p. 16). Jennings et al. (2020) draw on Mike White (2009) to explain how 'creative arts interventions in healthcare settings help to build relationships, maintain resilience, create more comfortable and user-friendly clinical environments, and support holistic approaches to care' (Jennings et al. 2020: p. 189). Arts activities are a means of 'nurturing and sustaining meaningful human relationships' in support of individual and social health and well-being (Ibid, p. 3). The development of arts and health as a field—more precisely the development of arts-based therapies—owes much to Moreno & Moreno's development of psychodrama and psychotherapy (Moreno and Moreno 1972). Moving away from 'talking therapies' their ideas for therapy were instead based on a 'pre-verbal ability to act' through certain issues using dramatic techniques such as role-play, especially in situations where one might be less able 'to articulate [issues] verbally' (Wasylko and Stickley 2003: p. 444).

Similar applications of arts-based approaches to support health and well-being have continued to grow and develop in a wide range of areas, as reflected in the UK government APPG report *Creative Health* (2017). The report presents substantial evidence that participation in the arts can be beneficial for mental and physical health, recovery, and well-being. Baxter and Low (2017) argue for a deeper understanding of the impact that social factors such as economic disadvantage, environmental pollution, and geographic and psychological isolation can have on health outcomes. From their perspective, applied theatre interventions into health should specifically aim to address social inequalities, political structures, and other contextual factors, as well as support well-being through participation. This particular argument is linked to those that inter-relate art with culture, specifically in a way that positions arts as a driver of culture creation and often enrichment.

Art and Culture

The development of arts and health as a field has proliferated in the last decade, to the point at which the same question of whether participation in the arts positively affects our health has been asked in wider contexts. As a result, the way that the arts enhance, produce, shape, and develop culture is increasingly under the microscope. For some, the arts and culture are somewhat synonymous, and general investment in both is theorised to lead to improved health (Aston 2014). The Arts Council England (ACE) has produced case studies and reports aplenty that point to the positive outcomes the arts and culture have on the well-being of the public (see: http://www. artscouncil.org.uk/wellbeing). Meanwhile, the Arts Council of Ireland (ACI) have highlighted the need to support artists, for instance through the task force report *Life Worth Living* (2020) which maps out a recovery path for arts and culture. The general assumption is that arts support culture, and by extension support health and wellbeing, and so society must support arts and artists to keep up their work in creating culture and supporting the health and wellbeing of the society.

Belfiore and Bennett (2008) point out that this assumption is in some ways ignorant to the fact that art and culture have been uneasy bedfellows. They cite Plato's *Republic* (2007) in particular as an indication of how the arts have been historically perceived as something harmful for a society to engage in. For Belfiore and Bennett (2008), the social and cultural impact of the arts is not really 'the point' of art, and they are highly critical of arts practice that is instrumentalised for a particular—non-arts based—benefit.[3] This view limits the potential of the arts to exist in other categories beyond, say, the entertainment industry, or as an elitist pursuit of higher understanding through aesthetic consumption, and so on. In short, this idea removes art from the everyday and places it in a higher category of experience than everyday reality. This notion is particularly uncomfortable concerning participatory arts characterised by a relational aesthetic of care (Thompson 2015; Nicholson 2017; Stuart Fisher and Thompson 2020).

Viewpoints characterised by an aesthetic of care directly contradict the statement that '[t]he aesthetic encounter, above all, is an individual subjective experience' (Belfiore and Bennett 2008: p. 6) which is the central logic behind arguments against assessing art by its broader social and cultural impact. When aesthetics are co-constructed relationally, in process, and with care, it is clear that the effects of arts activities are never solely determined by one single individual. Pressingly, seeing the fundamental aspect of art and aesthetics as subjective individual interpretation serves to only create and maintain art as an elitist pastime. Those who take the position asserted by Belfiore and Bennett (2008) would have art ring-fenced by gatekeepers who are the only ones who might access the deeper mysteries of its practice and understanding. I argue that shifting the appreciation of aesthetics to the relational caring encounter is an essential step to democratising art, and the cultures created, sustained, and enriched by arts practice. In this way, I purposefully align this study, and the direction of drama and nursing as an interdisciplinary field within the emerging field of care aesthetics (Thompson 2015; Nicholson 2017; Thompson 2023).

This study sits within the realm of nursing education, which in the UK is conducted at universities and regulated by a code of practice (NMC 2018). What I hope

---

[3] We are returning here to the argument of "art for art's sake" which bubbles under the surface of this study.

to illustrate is that applying drama to this context for PCN serves a particular purpose, with a method that is easily shared, and the impacts of which affect practitioners' ability to perform care—by extension, enhancing the experiences of those being 'cared for'. In many ways, the purpose of my work is the shared discovery encountered when working across the disciplines of drama and nursing. However, researchers from both fields raise some well-founded concerns about how a shared purpose privileges one or the other. This is a position that demarcates the field of arts and health, and in particular, the field of medical humanities where the power imbalance between the fields of medicine and the humanities is perceived to be significant. It is this perceived imbalance that drives disciplinary territorialism and makes meaningful interdisciplinary and cross-cultural dialogue difficult.

Medical Humanities

The medical humanities are an interdisciplinary field which positions medical disciplines alongside the disciplines comprising the humanities. Bates et al. (2014) describe publications and projects that define themselves as medical humanities as far back as 1979 and illustrate the diasporic growth of the practice from that point onwards. For Mermikides (2020), the 'shared preoccupation' for medicine and the humanities—in her example, drama and performance—is the human, and one step further, what is humane (p. 1). In a strange sense, the medical humanities are at once broader and narrower as a distinct field and/or discipline than that of arts and health as described earlier. Although the two fields share similar traits, and certainly overlap one another, the medical humanities are more difficult to define. This could be because work defined within the medical humanities often involves very contextual and project-specific approaches, without an agreed set of general principles or practices. Moreover, both terms that make up the definition, i.e., medicine and human— are ones which, although specific, are not universally defined as independent terms in either field. The confusion with this definition grows exponentially when the two terms are brought together (Bates et al. 2014; Clift and Camic 2016; Mermikides 2020). One unifying principle of various projects within the spectrum of the medical humanities is a process of interdisciplinarity, although this process takes on many faces.

Though the broad scope of the term medical humanities might be difficult to define, specific practices and dialogues across the disciplines have more promise to be clearly expressed, delineated, and shared. These aspects might be understood as general principles for work defined within the medical humanities. Bates et al. (2014) argue against defining the field as 'a clear-cut definition could remove the diversity of approach that makes the medical humanities so appealing in the first place' (p. 4). It is indeed hard to define the medical humanities as a catch-all term, though the contextual and specific practices which make up the medical humanities are more readily definable. I argue, in tentative agreement with Bates et al, that following these contextual paths and defining them would in turn define the medical humanities. I disagree that this would then limit the potential of medical humanities.

Though there may be many general principles, this profligacy of contextual features simply reflects the dynamic and effusive interplay between the two disciplines. Definition need not reduce the diversity of the medical humanities, but resisting clear definitions does restrict how the practices can be transposed, adopted, and practiced.

I argue that the majority of the unease with defining the medical humanities (and in a smaller way arts and health) stems from an anxiety that once defined the perceived 'aura' of certain artistic approaches reduces. In simple terms, this position asserts that if we define and explain art through non-artist approaches we lose its apparently immeasurable ephemerality. In turn, those who can navigate and interpret the less easily measurable features of arts and humanities are no longer just 'the experts'. Reason and Rowe (2017) argue that 'the death of the expert' has had a profound cultural effect on Western societies and has validated individuals to reject experts outright, often meaning opinion stands in for evidence. This makes claiming the cultural benefits of arts more fraught than ever for many folks. To grossly oversimply, this means that assertions made about what art 'can do' may be dismissed as anecdotes rather than evidence, with expert voices drowned out in the cultural fog of disbelief. Along similar lines, Clift et al. (2010) and Clift and Camic (2016), rightly ask whether arts practices that state beneficial outcomes sustain participation as 'an elitist luxury available only to the already advantaged' (Clift et al. 2010: p. 8). The dichotomy this produces is the need for experts to produce evidence we can support and trust on the one hand, and democratising the arts to be for everyone to contribute towards and to take part in on the other. For many researchers, this debate means they are uneasy about relinquishing control of their discipline and/or approaches, and they feel defining the field of medical humanities is a part of relinquishing this control. In short, the unease to establish generalised principles can be used as a way to maintain a disciplinary territorialism that ill-serves the development of the field. For me, much of the 'aura' of these approaches is rooted in the notion of the arts as a fundamentally subjective experience. Though I agree that this makes it hard to suggest one person can objectively 'know' more than another about that experience, there are people who simply have more *experience* of the subjective experience of art. These are the experts who should carry more *caché* in debates. As such, though I disagree on whether or not to define the medical humanities as part of relinquishing control over the field, I agree with Bates et al.'s (2014) positioning of medical humanities as a 'multi-discipline'. I also interject that art is far more an inter-subjective (and intra-subjective) experience than simply a subjective one. This allows the inclusion of specific and rich offshoots as a collection and accumulation of subjective experience, as seen for example in Mermikides' (2020) exploration of 'medical performance' as a distinctly contemporary phenomenon within the arena of medical humanities. It is in these offshoots that the richness of contextual and specific practices and experiences come to construct the medical humanities, which by themselves could easily be defined in general terms as a process of open dialogue across the fields of medicine and the humanities. This expansion of the field points to relationality—the inter-subjective experience—as an essential factor in aesthetic experiences.

This study is not explicitly positioned within the medical humanities, but I cannot ignore its implicit place within the medical humanities spectrum as well as the argument for a medical humanities that this study presents by its very existence. Although there are many shared and resonant features this study moves away from the medical as the central focus of healthcare. Instead, this study is aligned with the PCNF (McCormack and McCance 2010). As such the focus is on the role of the nurse and nursing-specific care. By aligning with the PCNF, this study also turns attention to the concept of personhood over humanity, or as Mermikides (2020) points out, the humane, which is perhaps closer to the notion of person-centredness. That said, this study at its heart does ask whether drama participation can enhance the humanistic practices of PCN. This is a crucial difference that the PCNF is not a medical framework, it is a nursing-specific framework. PCN is in many ways a response to the over-medicalization of nursing, and as such much of the key work usually associated with the humanities within medical humanities is already happening, or decades established. This frees up the study to look at specific conceptual and practical aspects of PCN through the prism of drama participation. The distinct practices and principles of drama participation have a long history and a complex relationship to notions of education and applications for utilitarian purposes beyond being applied to medicine and health.

Theatre in Education and Applied Drama

Theatre in education (TIE) as a term encompasses a wide range of drama practices found in educational settings. Anthony Jackson (2007) describes the emergence of the paradigm in the UK in the 1960s. Helen Nicholson (2011) explains that a key feature of theatre and performance in education is in how it challenges dominant Western ideas of how knowledge is understood and cultivated. For Nicholson (2011), TIE demonstrates that 'knowledge is not fixed, but always mobile, fluid, created and recreated through dialogue and in relation to others', and that 'understanding is not always articulated in language' (p. 10). TIE has been directly and indirectly influenced by ideas such as Dewey's experiential learning (1916), Freire's Pedagogy of the Oppressed (2000), Boal's development of Freire's ideas in his Theatre of the Oppressed (TO; Boal 1998), Vygotsky's notion of the Zone of Proximal Development (1978), Gardener's Multiple Intelligences (1993), Kolb's learning cycle (1984), Johnston's notion of making theatre from everyday life (1998), and more.

In a similar vein to arts and health and medical humanities, TIE is an expansive field. The broad scope of pedagogical applications within the spectrum of TIE alone illustrates this. As Jackson and Vine introduces and briefly summarises, these areas are Applied drama, theatre for development, TO, Educational theatre, young people's theatre, Children's theatre and Theatre for young audiences, youth theatre, theatre education, set play workshops and/or play days, museum theatre, process drama and/or drama in education, drama therapy, and simulation gaming (Jackson and Vine 2013: p. 10–13). Nicholson mostly situates TIE in educational environments involving young people where the use of performance encourages 'young people to find points of connection between lived experience and theatrical representation' (Nicholson 2011: p. 5). Whereas Jackson & Vine situates TIE more openly as an approach that 'seeks to harness the techniques and imaginative potency of theatre in the service of education' (2013: p. 5). Both these positions capture the essence of TIE and also illustrate the early development of applied drama in what I feel are distinct but complementary modalities.

Applied drama can be defined as a social practice that uses drama to, among so much more, challenge accepted practices, remake social realities, and promote active roles in citizenship (Nicholson 2005; Hughes et al. 2011; O'Connor and Anderson 2015). O'Connor & Anderson cite Goffman's theory of the 'dramaturgy of everyday life' as inciting the performative turn, where interactions are a performance of a self in public (Goffman 1990; O'Connor and Anderson 2015). This was an influential turn which led to the application of concepts for producing productions on stage to explore—and often try to improve—aspects of people's everyday lives. This 'everyday performance' was foundational to Boal in TO (Boal 1998), derived through Freire's dialogical pedagogy and pedagogy of the oppressed (Freire 1998, 2000; Freire et al. 2004). Boal's work uses theatre to reveal the everyday oppressions communities face and to work through these using performance strategies (Boal 1998). As described above, practitioners such as Jackson expanded upon existing educational drama approaches using Boal's work, creating more democratic and dialogic approaches to a wide range of pedagogical spaces (Jackson 2007). Applied drama as a field borrows deeply from these educational approaches and provides an interactive pedagogical methodology that resonates with espoused notions of PCN such as authenticity, morality, reflexivity, and embodiment. As with TIE, the scope of applied drama is an effusive one, which is difficult to pin down with any definitional certainty. To avoid perceived restrictions to practice, many call for considering applied drama as an ecology of practice rather than a specific and specialised 'field'.

The Ecology of Applied Drama Practice

Applied drama is often considered as an umbrella practice or as Hughes & Nicholson describe, '[a]n ecology of practices [that] promises to hold divergent and critical perspectives in conversation, enabling connections to be found' (2016: p. 3). Although many drama-based practices sit comfortably within this ecology, others have been less considered. For instance, 'whilst Boal's approaches are probably the most influential in the field (Babbage 2004) Stanislavski's approaches to acting and actor training are less commonly associated with applied drama' (Jennings et al. 2020: p. 195). Speculatively, this might in part be due to a preconception of the place of acting and the actor in drama studies through concepts such as Michael Kirby's 'non-acting' (1972) and Hans Lehmann's 'postdramatic theatre' (2006) which amongst others both challenge the primacy of acting as the *modus operandi* of drama and theatre. It may also be due to a historical conception of Stanislavskian methods as closely aligned with what Nicholson identifies as 'pure' drama concerned with 'abstract and theoretical' notions of the aesthetic, rather than applied drama which explores 'using theoretical models to solve practical problems' beyond the stage (Nicholson 2005, p. 5–6).

Nicholson draws attention to the distinctions between 'pure' and 'applied' to highlight and criticise the problematic and often exclusionary divide that can exist in the field. Hughes and Nicholson's (2016) concept of applied drama as an 'ecology of practices' highlights a perception that the practical methods adopted by applied drama can access the aesthetic through—for instance—affect theory. Perhaps reductively, applied drama does not have to be 'shit theatre' that serves a simple purpose. At the same time, 'pure' drama is increasingly open to including 'low' forms of aesthetics and a 'DIY' attitude (Daniels 2014, 2015) and is more readily inclusive of political and social purpose (see, for example, the theatre makers *Sh!t Theatre*). Considering the methods suggested by Stanislavski aside from their formal presentation (i.e., a 'beautifully' and realistically acted play, often described as 'naturalism'), I argue that his approach is more suited to use as a model 'to solve practical problems' (Nicholson 2005: p. 6) than previously thought.

Although it seems like the central tenet of the term applied drama, many practitioners and theorists feel deep unease with the idea of applying drama to solve particular issues (Freebody et al. 2018). The central premise of the debate is whether applied drama only has value if it has a 'real' effect on existing problems, or whether value stems from factors beyond utility. The debate of what—and often who—applied drama is for can be a divisive topic. A key fault line in this argument is how to measure and understand the success, value, and impact of applied theatre work (Belfiore and Bennett 2008; Reason and Rowe 2017; Freebody et al. 2018). This is often tempered with the added difficulty from grant funders to achieve certain goals which some think undermines or ignores more meaningful goals (Snyder-Young 2018). Some take this criticism further to suggest that policymakers and funders often set goals that suit their idea of a successful outcome for a participant. For example, Low (2020) critically reflects on her past project which attempted to measure behaviour change as an unwitting part of 'a neoliberal push to impose predetermined outcomes on a particular group of participants' (p. 15). There is a strong push from some researchers to ensure that applied drama projects in all their variety have their success, value, and impact measured in applied drama oriented ways. This has grown into something of a disquiet for some applied drama researchers to the idea of welcoming research methods from outside of the discipline (Freebody et al. 2018). This study purposefully argues against the notion of excluding external methods from applied drama research. Instead, I hope to use methods and approaches that are complementary to and translated across both fields. Moreover, I find no qualm in basing the success, value, and impact of the study on metrics familiar to PCN, and dismiss the idea that this in some way diminishes the applied drama-based impact of the work. Likewise, I refuse to shy away from presenting the outcomes in a drama-based perspective to PCN environs.[4] I firmly argue that applied drama needs to recognise its place as a fundamentally interdisciplinary approach. Perhaps this is easier to acknowledge for me in this project, as the profession to which drama is being applied in my context has an explicit code of practice like nursing does in the UK (NMC 2018). Further, the goals of PCN are more aligned with arts and humanities concepts of success than, say, medical science. One way to find collective verbiage for research across disciplines (including nursing and drama) is by using and combining a variety of approaches and evidence, to create a 'cumulative construction of evidence through the weaving of multiple strands' (Reason and Rowe 2017: p. 8). One of the key strands to position this study is how applied drama has enhanced, and effected healthcare.

Applied drama's transformative social potential has been used in healthcare to address 'fluid and subtle social determinants of health' (Baxter and Low 2017: p. 40). Applied drama in healthcare advocates for an inter-subjective, social, and inter-relational approach to care rather than an objective, abstract, model of clinical medical care. This broadly reflects the distinction between a 'social model' and a 'medical model' of health. Emma Brodzinski (2010) examines the specific ways in which theatre has been used and has engaged with notions of health. These include ways in which theatre has been performed in health institutions, how theatre has been used for health education, theatre as a means of accessing health and citizenship, and theatre as an influence for developing health care simulation.

Role play and simulation are a 'a core element of health care training globally [...] [o]ne common approach is to use actors to play patients in role plays (known as 'standardised patients' or 'patient actors'), an internationally established practice since the 1960s (Barrows 1993)' (Jennings et al. 2020: p. 190). The use of such patient actors allows healthcare students to simulate the practitioner–patient relationship and practice their skills with them in a more consequence-free environment. This approach has become crucial to the assessment of students and practitioners of medicine and nursing. For instance, all UK-based health professionals must demonstrate their clinical skills through evaluation processes like the Objective Structured Clinical Examination (OSCE), which includes elements of simulation and role play. Another example, as previously mentioned, is Mermikides' (2020) application of drama approaches with nurses, aimed at the affective, emotional, and empathetic aspects of nursing care. Empathy features in many practices where drama is applied to healthcare. Some (Reeves et al. 2021) have used elements of Stanislavskian actor training to help nurses to attend to emotions and empathy. One particular—and for me contentious—method is 'emotion memory'. A critique of emotion memory and the potential pitfalls of using it in a health context are presented in the next chapter. Before this, a specific and common way that drama relates and applies to is simulation practice.

---

[4] Indeed, I have purposefully presented using performative means at nursing conferences, sharing the thrust of the value of the approach as something embodied, experienced, and created live and in the moment. This has included "acting for" nursing audiences, as well as inviting these audiences to act with me, to feel it for themselves.

Healthcare Simulation

Simulation training often involves the aim of developing specific clinical skills and providing clinical experience without patient risk (Lateef 2010). There are many types of simulation, and they are often seen as positive learning experiences. However, some cause stress and anxiety, like the OSCE exam (Fidment 2012). There is evidence that when designed to address more than a single clinical skill in isolation simulation can enhance clinical skills alongside other aspects of competence, such as decision making, holistic care, and critical thinking (Lazzari 2011; Victor et al. 2017). Taylor et al (2021) suggest clinical placements can be simulated and achieve a similar, if not, more effective pedagogical outcome than traditional learning placements. Healthcare simulation often involves various technologies as well as elements that could be described as theatrical (McAllister et al. 2013b; Reid-Searl et al. 2017).

Jennings et al. (2020) argue that though manikins 'for medical simulation are increasingly sophisticated, automated, and technically specific [...] a reliance on robotic mannequins can reinforce mechanistic paradigms of treatment, as against more holistic approaches' (p. 191). Tizzard-Kleister and Jennings (2020) reflect that 'replacing the human patient with a mannequin' in SRP and throughout nursing education may contribute to nurses seeing their care as transactional and dehumanised, reinforcing 'perceptions of patients as passive and inert' (Tizzard-Kleister and Jennings 2020: p.74; Jansen et al. 2009; Ellis et al. 2015). Moreover, experience and expertise in the theatrical nature of simulation is often lacking, restricting the potential of the approach as a pedagogical experience beyond skill acquisition and demonstration. Instead of simple skill acquisition, SRP should strive 'to create immersive events or situations that enable a student to spontaneously respond in a controlled environment that nevertheless reflects their anticipated work experience' (Arrighi et al. 2018: p. 89). There is still a great need for more simulation practices and approaches that aim to enhance interpersonal skills like teamwork, leadership, communication, and more alongside clinical skills (Siassakos et al. 2011; Hallenbeck 2012; Levett-Jones and Lapkin 2014).

It is a widely held belief that drama applied to healthcare simulation and SRP in particular stimulates creative and unique learning in a 'safe and standardised environment' (Wheeler and Mcnelis 2014: p. 260–261; Wilson et al. 2015; McCullough 2012). In some cases, drama has been applied to simulations to address issues such as the stress caused by simulated exams (Fidment 2012; Jennings et al. 2020). McAllister et al. (2013b) point out that in simulations 'students may realise the setting is artificial and fail to fully engage', suggesting the application of drama would be helpful to increase student engagement (McAllister et al. 2013b: p. 1453). Brodzinski (2010) states that often students are 'painfully aware of the false nature of the scenarios' (p. 123–4), advocating for more applications from drama to enliven the process and enhance the believability of the scenarios explored. Jennings et al. (2020) highlight the studies of Bach and Grant (2017) and Gault et al. (2017) in advocating for SRP that 'focus on kindness, respect, and compassion' (p. 191). McEvoy and Duffy (2008) concur and urge for SRP that takes account of 'the person as a whole' and to explore 'the interrelationship of body, mind, and spirit' in nursing care through SRP (p. 414).

Arts approaches have been applied to achieve this (Yakhforoshha et al. 2017; Tilbrook et al. 2017), where drama specifically has been used for enhancing what de Oliveira et al. (2015) calls 'psychological fidelity'—the felt authenticity in the encounter for the participant in a simulated situation. Often, simulations involving drama serve to deepen the fidelity of the interaction between clinician and patient (Buxton 2011). The application of drama to enhance this fidelity has provided a process through which participants can develop 'creative and critical-reflexive skills' (de Oliveira et al. 2015: p. 54). One aim of my work demonstrated through this book is to highlight the potential for drama approaches to be applied to SRP to deepen the fidelity of the scenario (in realism, or psychological 'authenticity') and to find a way to come closer to feeling 'real', but to go beyond that and provide something extraordinary. I hope to show how drama can help SRP as a pedagogical method to look beyond simply representing the real situations of healthcare practices, to instead explore how to use that reality as a basis for experiencing and navigating deep and complex situations and questions. If SRP is to play a meaningful part in developing the workforce of tomorrow, we cannot be satisfied with approaches that simply represent the current reality. Drama has the potential to aid learners in holding the real world and the performed world together in the same moment. Therefore, Drama applied to SRP can not only help students to engage with psychological authenticity as de Oliveira et al. (2015) suggest, but it can also provide crucial methods and skills for healthcare students and professionals to overcome unforeseen challenges through cultivating skills to better perform sympathetic presence. To begin to see the potential of drama to enhance SRP in ways beyond *mise en scene*, promoting psychological fidelity, or increased realism, it is worth turning attention to ways drama has been applied to nursing education more broadly.

Drama in Nursing Education

Though arts and health as a field have seen recent attention for its potential to revolutionise healthcare (APPG 2017; Fancourt and Finn 2019), the breadth and variety of the field mean specific features of particular disciplines—such as drama—have been under-considered in the main literature on arts and health (Fancourt 2017). For Noonan et al. (2016) 'engagement with the creative arts in nursing and midwifery education offers one route to explore, expand, and enhance students' non-normative ethics and values that underpin the sustained delivery of person-centred compassionate care' (p. 309). In Noonan et al.'s (2016) chapter on this, drama is not a subject they explore. Some reviews have sought to bring together and make sense of the place of drama in the field of arts and health in the last 10 years (Perry et al. 2011; Wilson et al. 2015; Arveklev et al. 2015).

Drama has historically been used for its educational potential in collaboration with some aspects of health, such as healthcare simulation (Barrows 1993; Brodzinski 2010), however, this is often limited to employing drama students or professional actors in the role of the simulated patient (Anderson et al. 2010; Aldridge 2017). The application of drama approaches to enhance the performance of simulated patients tackles problems such as patient dehumanisation through over-reliance on medical mannequins in simulation (Jansen et al. 2009; McAllister et al. 2013a; Ellis et al. 2015). Some projects have sought to increase the fidelity of these patients in SRP by improving the realism of the performance through the inclusion of drama students or professional actors (Burton et al. 2015; Jacobs and van Jaarsveldt 2016). Though these approaches might enhance the fidelity of a simulation, they neglect the potential that using the same techniques might have for enhancing healthcare students' interactive skills (Goodwin and Deady 2013; Macneill et al. 2014, 2016). Evidence is clearly building that applying drama to SRP builds practical healthcare professional skills (Dickinson et al. 2016; Lawrence and Wier 2018; Jennings et al. 2020).

There are some projects which have engaged healthcare students directly in drama workshops with various objectives and outcomes. For instance, some examples are; enhancing students' ethical thinking (McCullough 2012), encouraging students and staff to engage in holistic approaches to providing care (Willson 2006), developing an awareness of how status and power affect everyday interactions for students (Taylor and Taylor 2017), enhancing practitioner creativity (Dümenci and Keçeci 2014), supporting students' ability to reflect in and on action (Arveklev et al. 2020), and using student-led approaches to developing inter-professional collaboration and advocacy (Kyle et al. 2023). Some approaches like these focus on the patient perspective as a specific learning point (Kooken and Kerr 2018). In the connected work of Lepp (2002), Ekebergh et al. (2004) and Arveklev et al. (2018a, b) drama helps to access other's 'life-worlds', putting 'students in different caring situations, with their patients and their perspective in focus' (Lepp 2002: p. 3). In this way, drama has been used to help make the patient's perspective explicit to nursing students. Directly engaging nursing students with drama workshops seems to lead to a wider variety of outcomes in unique and often powerful experiences.

However, there is room for more ideas from applied drama to be included in these approaches, especially in roles that involve more patient interaction (Jennings et al. 2020). Moreover, drama approaches can be applied to known issues in new ways. For instance, tackling the possibility of patient dehumanisation by attempting to anthropomorphise medical mannequins to become 'human patients' (Bennett 2010; Bogost 2012; Wharram 2014). This is particularly innovative through applied puppetry techniques (Smith 2015; Tizzard-Kleister and Jennings 2020; Hulkko and Laakkonen 2022). Applied drama used in healthcare simulation has the potential to facilitate a more critical and creative interactive learning method, where power dynamics are equalised through dialogue between facilitators and students who teach and learn from one another. This might be deeply resonant for PCN in terms of helping to understand personhood in a more practical sense. Specifically, students can come to understand how to express their personhood. They can then understand how others express their personhood and find ways to make interactions with them a mutual exchange. As Brodzinski highlights 'engaging in theatre practice may serve to enable participants to realise their potential as healthy citizens and develop the voice they already have as a means of expressing their personhood' (2010: p. 89–90). There are few examples of drama-based interventions in health-care which specifically focus on the concepts explained throughout PCN such as personhood (Kontos et al. 2010; Dingwall et al. 2017; Boersma et al. 2019), and those that do, do not use other resonant concepts from the PCNF, such as sympathetic presence.

Jennings et al. (2020) explore how '[t]here has been little crossover to date between the specific practice of healthcare simulation and the broader social practices of applied drama' (p. 190). Whilst Souza et al. (2015) presents compelling arguments for the use of 'dramatisation techniques as a pedagogical strategy' for nurses 'to reflect on their professional praxis' (p. 3547). What is often lacking is an articulation of what these techniques might be. There are also very few examples which acknowledge the field of applied drama unless these are written by applied drama theorists or practitioners themselves (one good example is Reeves et al. 2021). This suggests that perhaps the long histories, established theories, and tried-and-tested methodologies of this field are not known to health-based staff who take part in and lead these interventions. I hope the irony of this is clear, namely that some of those leading the application of drama into nursing are less aware of the field and ecology of 'applied' drama. I also wish to make it clear that this is not a judgemental observation, particularly as I openly acknowledge my ignorance of applied drama before undertaking this doctoral study. This is an observation which highlights the necessity of the relevant expertise from both fields to be equally present and represented. I am critical of research about how drama has been applied to nursing (and, albeit more rarely, research on how nursing has been applied to drama), that does not include authors with expertise from both disciplines.

Jennings et al. (2020) state how 'applied drama interventions that do engage with health care training seek to support the development of creativity and empathy in general terms' (p. 190). This resonates with how the medical humanities seeks to humanise medicine (White 2009; Baxter and Low 2017; Fancourt 2017). What is rarer are projects which tap into 'applied drama techniques to address specific problems in the performance of health care' (Jennings et al. 2020: 190). Though not explicitly an applied drama project, Mermikides' *Careful* (2020) is an example of a project which does just that, as it involves applications of drama workshops and performance practice for nurses. Approaches like these 'have sought to narrow the gap between these potentially complementary performative techniques', the ecology of applied drama, and nursing (Jennings et al. 2020: 190). One project which stands out in this regard is a project created by the theatre company *Clod Ensemble,* called 'Performing Medicine' (APPG 2017; Willson and Jaye 2017). The 'Performing Medicine' project involves performance workshops with healthcare professionals, where they learn different skills and practices from dancers, actors, visual artists, and more. This includes the 'Circle of Care' model, which focus on 'nonverbal communication, self-care, spatial awareness, and appreciation of the person with an emphasis on understanding the perspectives and contexts of others' (Willson and Jaye 2017: p. 643).

There have been some examples of designed drama-based interventions with nursing students that have enabled 'students to experiment with different roles' offering 'an opportunity to explore their own individual vulnerability in a safe environment' (Arveklev et al. 2015:p. e13). The work of Susanna Arveklev (Arveklev et al. 2015; Arveklev et al. 2018a, b, 2020) exemplifies an interdisciplinary approach using drama to enhance nursing education. Arveklev et al.'s (2015) review of the literature on drama and nursing identified three resonant themes between the examples from the field: 'the framing', 'the objective', and 'the embodiment'. The idea of embodiment in this particular case resonates with Nolan's (2009) ideas on how embodiment creates agency and culture through the performing of gestures. In their intervention involving drama workshops with nursing students Arveklev et al. (2018a) identified that '[d]rama provided an opportunity to practice dialogues with patients and highlighted the importance of focusing on the patient's narrative and to listen actively' (p. 64). Meanwhile, they suggest 'to focus future studies on curriculum development' to explore more ways drama might enhance nursing education in a more sustained and integrated way (Ibid: p. 65). I wholeheartedly agree with this conclusion.

In 2020, Arveklev et al reported on a project involving 'forum-play', an approach adding elements of play to Boal's 'Forum Theatre' (1998).[5] In this example, 'ethical problems became clearer and the situations easier to understand when they were dramatised and reflected on' (Arveklev et al. 2020: p. 4). Reeves and Neilson (2018) use forum theatre to improve interactive skills of nursing students' in the context of palliative care. Forum theatre is—relatively speaking—fairly frequently used when applying drama to nursing. For instance, Middlewick et al. (2012) used forum theatre to explore the 'art of communication' with nursing students, meanwhile, Bogue et al. (2017) adapted Boal's forum theatre approach to use what they call 'touch-tag theatre'—which removes the singular protagonist and joker to encourage a communal approach—with postgraduate nursing students to explore emotional intelligence.

Alison Reeves and Sue Neilson across several publications report on the outcomes of using forum theatre as an approach to enhance learning on dealing with sensitive communication issues, for example, the death of a child (Reeves and Neilson 2018; Neilson and Reeves 2019; Reeves et al. 2021). Many who use approaches such as these advocate for integrating these approaches more into nursing curricula. Bogue et al. (2017) specifically advocate lengthening applied drama interventions in nursing education, as well as training nursing staff in the practice so they might use it in clinical workplaces. Highlighting that for their participants 'most of their challenges are actually experienced with other members of staff rather

---

[5] Forum Theatre is an approach developed by Boal (1998) and is well-known and very commonly used in applied drama practices. To summarise, the approach involves a group performing a scene depicting a protagonist having a difficult time. The scene is then played again, and the audience is invited by a *compère* (called the Joker) to pause the action at any time, replace an actor, and attempt to improvise a different way forward. It aims to help spectators break through their passivity to become what Boal calls "spect-actors". To see more on how this approach has been used in nursing see: Reeves et al. (2021)

than patients' (Bogue et al. 2017: p. 113). Ekebergh et al. (2004) report on the development of the DRACAR model, an acronym abbreviated from the description drama caring and reflection in nursing education model. They describe their project where drama workshops are delivered alongside other nursing teaching to bridge the theory-praxis gap. In their sessions students take part in 'role-play, forum-theatre, and nursing-play' to explore communication skills and more (Ekebergh et al. 2004: p. 625). As Jennings et al. (2020) highlight, projects like these 'could potentially begin to bridge the gap between arts in health practices and conventional health care simulation, and subsequently seed the nascent field of drama in nursing' (p. 191).

Actor Training, Simulated Patients, and Nursing Education

Although a growing majority of drama-based interventions in healthcare focus on the work of Boal (1998), particularly his use of 'Forum Theatre' (Ekebergh et al. 2004; Arveklev et al. 2018a, b; Neilson and Reeves 2019), one of the more traditionally common applications is in facilitating and enhancing the use of standardised patients, usually actors playing the role of patients in an SRP (Barrows 1993; Loth et al. 2015). Arrighi et al. (2018) in particular criticise the lack of training for those performing the role of standardised patients, suggesting the use of actor training through the work of Constantin Stanislavski (1990) to support and enhance the performance of these roles. They identify two main strengths that this approach can address; '(1) the creation of well-rounded characters developed from real-life observation […] and (2) the development of improvisation skills and intuitive awareness of the best and truest impulse' (Arrighi et al. 2018: p. 90). I argue that these same outcomes—and some other potentially unexpected ones—may also occur for healthcare students when taught actor training methods. Goodwin and Deady (2013) agree and argue that teaching nursing students the 'specifics of The System and The Method would advance lessons and skills learned through role play, allowing practitioners to enhance the levels of empathy they display' (p. 131). However, they are working through more traditional forms of empathy, and draw from Stanislavski's ideas on 'emotional memory' to encourage practitioners to create a 'sincerity of emotion' (Stanislavski 1961: p. 34; cited in Goodwin and Deady 2013).

Aligned with Jennings et al. (2020) and the PCNF (McCormack and McCance 2010) this study disputes the use of emotional memory and its counterpart empathy in educating nurses using drama-based methods. Instead, I argue for the use of approaches from Stanislavski's 'Method of Physical Action' (MoPA) in conjunction with sympathetic presence. The concept of 'emotion memory' and how it has been applied to nursing education and simulation will be specifically critiqued as potentially problematic in the next chapter. It is argued that a focus on Stanislavski's MoPA, where actions determine actors' character and behaviour (Benedetti 1998; Carnicke 2010), is more suitable to use as a technical approach to teach similar skills. This is particularly pertinent when considering that the impulsion to use one's emotional reserves as frequently seen in empathetic approaches may be a chief cause of anxiety, which leads to an aversion to risk-taking. These issues will be expounded and untangled in the following two chapters.

References

Aldridge MD (2017) Standardized patients portraying parents in paediatric end-of-life simulation. Clin Simul Nurs 13(7):338–342

All-Party Parliamentary Group (APPG) (2017) Creative health: The arts for health and wellbeing. All-Party Parliamentary Group, London. http://www.artshealthandwellbeing.org.uk/appg-inquiry/Publications/Creative_Health_Inquiry_Report_2017_-_Second_Edition.pdf. Accessed 30 Oct 2018

Anderson M, Holmes TL, LeFlore JL, Nelson KA, Jenkins T (2010) Standardized patients in educating student nurses: one school's experience. Clin Simul Nurs 6(2):61–66

Arrighi G, Irvine C, Joyce B, Kristi Haracz K (2018) Reimagining 'role' and 'character': an approach to acting training for role-play simulation in the tertiary education setting. Appl Theatr Res 6(2):89–106

Arts Council Ireland (ACI) (2020) Life worth living report. Arts Council Ireland. Life Worth Living: The Report of the Arts and Culture Recovery Taskforce | The Arts Council | An Chomhairle Ealaíon—Accessed 4 Feb 2021

Arveklev SH, Wigert H, Berg L, Burton B, Lepp M (2015) The use and application of drama in nursing education — an integrative review of the literature. Nurse Educ Today 35(7):e12–e17

Arveklev SH, Berg L, Wigert H, Morrison-Helme M, Lepp M (2018a) Nursing students experiences of learning about nursing through drama. Nurse Educ Pract 28:60–65

Arveklev SH, Berg L, Wigert H, Morrison-Helme M, Lepp M (2018b) Learning about conflict and conflict management through drama in nursing education. J Nurs Educ 57(4):209–216

Arveklev S, Wigert H, Berg L, Lepp M (2020) Specialist nursing students' experiences of learning through drama in paediatric care. Nurse Educ Pract 43:1–6

Aston J (2014) Let's invest in real health. In: Arts Council England's create: a journal of perspectives on the value of art & Culture. Manchester, Arts Council England, pp 89–96

Babbage F (2004) Augusto Boal. Routledge, Abingdon

Bach S, Grant A (2017) Communication and interpersonal skills in nursing, 2nd edn. Sage, London

Barrows HS (1993) An overview of the uses of standardized patients for teaching and evaluating clinical skills. Acad Med 68(6):443–451

Bates V, Bleakley A, Goodman S (eds) (2014) Medicine, health and the arts : approaches to the medical humanities. Routledge, Abingdon

Baxter V, Low K (eds) (2017) Applied theatre: performing health and wellbeing. Bloomsbury, London

Belfast Health and Social Care Trust (2017) Patient and client feedback: an overview 2016–17. Belfast Health and Social Care Trust

Belfiore E, Bennett O (2008) The social impact of the arts. Palgrave Macmillan, London

Benedetti J (1998) Stanislavski and the actor. Methuen Drama, London

Bennett J (2010) Vibrant matter: a political ecology of things. Duke University Press, Durham

Bleakley A, Bligh J, Browne J (2011) Medical education for the future: identity, power and location. Springer, London

Boal A (1998) Theatre of the oppressed. Pluto Press, London

Boersma P, van Weert J, Lissenberg-Witte B, van Meijel B, Dröes R-M (2019) Testing the implementation of the Veder contact method: A theatre-based communication method in dementia care. Gerontologist 59(4):780–791

Bogost I (2012) Alien phenomenology, or what it's like to be a thing. University of Minnesota Press, Minnesota

Bogue R, Hahn M, Lynch C (2017) Rehearsing for life: applied theatre—a worthwhile pedagogic addition to those working and training in health and social care? The practitioner's perspective. Nurse Educ Today 51:112–113

Brodzinski E (2010) Theatre in health and care. Palgrave, Basingstoke

Brodzinski E (2014) Performance anxiety the relationship between social and aesthetic drama in medicine and health. In: Bates V, Bleakley A, Goodman S (eds) Medicine, health and the arts: approaches to the medical humanities. Routledge, Abingdon, pp 165–185

Burton B, Lepp M, Morrison M, O'Toole J (2015) Acting to manage conflict and bullying through evidence-based strategies. Springer, New York

Buxton B (2011) Interaction, unscripted: an effective use of drama to simulate the nurse-client relationship. J Psychol Nursing 49(5):28–32

Carnicke SM (2010) Stanislavsky's system: pathways for the actor. In: Hodge A (ed) Actor training. Routledge, Abingdon, pp 28–53

Clift S, Camic P (eds) (2016) Creative arts, health, and wellbeing: international perspectives on practice, policy, and research. Oxford University Press, Oxford

Clift S, Camic P, Daykin N (2010) The arts and global health inequalities. Arts Health : An international journal for research, policy, and practice 2:3–7

Cook NF, Brown D, O'Donnell D, McCance T, Dickson C, Tønnesen S, Dunleavy S, Lorber M, Falkenberg H, Byrne G, McCormack B (2022) The person-centred curriculum framework: a universal curriculum framework for person-centred healthcare practitioner education. Int Pract Dev J 12(4):1–11

Daniels R (2014) D.I.Y. University of Chichester, Chichester

Daniels R (2015) D.I.Y. too. University of Chichester, Chichester

de Oliveira SN, Prado MLD, Kempfer SS, Martini JG, Caravaca-Morera JA, Bernardi MC (2015) Experiential learning in nursing consultation education via clinical simulation with actors: action research. Nurse Educ Today 35(2):50–54

de Zulueta P (2013) Compassion in 21st century medicine: is it sustainable? Clinical Ethics 8(4):119–128

Dewey J (1916) Democracy and education: an introduction to the philosophy of education. Plain Label Books

Dewing J, McCormack B, McCance T (eds) (2021) Person-Centred nursing research: methodology, methods and outcomes. Springer, London

Dickinson T, Mawdsley D-L, Hanlon-Smith C (2016) Using drama to teach interpersonal skills: role of theatre in the education of health professionals and the opinions of nursing students involved in a post-show workshop. Ment Health Pract 19(8):22–24

Dingwall L, Fenton J, Kelly TB, Lee J (2017) Sliding doors: did drama-based inter-professional education improve the tensions round person-centred nursing and social care delivery for people with dementia: A mixed method exploratory study. Nurse Educ Today 51:1–7

Dümenci SB, Keçeci A (2014) Creative drama: can it be used in nursing education. Int J Hum Sci 11(2):1320–1326

Ekebergh M, Lepp M, Dahlberg K (2004) Reflective learning with Drama in nursing education—A Swedish attempt to overcome the theory praxis gap. Nurse Educ Today 24:622–628

Ellis DM, Brou R, King R, Tusa P (2015) Psychiatric simulation on a budget. Clin Simul Nurs 11(11):469–471

Fancourt D (2017) Arts in health: designing and researching interventions. Oxford University Press, Oxford

Fancourt D, Finn S (2019) What is the evidence on the role of the arts in improving health and well-being? WHO, Helsinki

Fidment S (2012) The objective structured clinical exam (OSCE): a qualitative study exploring the health care student's experience. Stud Engage Exp J 1(1):1–18

Francis R (2013) Report of the mid Staffordshire NHS Foundation Trust Public Inquiry: executive summary. The Stationery Office, London

Freebody K, Balfour M, Finneran M, Anderson M (eds) (2018) Applied theatre: understanding change. Springer, London

Freire P (1998) Pedagogy of freedom: ethics, democracy and civic courage. Rowman & Littlefield Publishers, Lanham, MD, Oxford

Freire P (2000) Pedagogy of the oppressed. Continuum, New York

Freire P, Barr RR, Freire P, Freire AMA (2004) Pedagogy of hope: reliving pedagogy of the oppressed. Continuum, London

Gardener H (1993) Multiple intelligences, Harper Collins: New York.

Gault I, Shapcott J, Luthi A, Reid G (2017) Communication in nursing and health care: a guide for compassionate practice. Sage, London

GMC (1993) Tomorrow's doctors: recommendations on undergraduate medical education. Education committee of the General Medical Council, London

Goffman E (1990) The presentation of self in everyday life. Penguin, London

Goodwin J, Deady R (2013) The art of mental health practice: the role of Drama in developing empathy. Perspect Psychiatr Care 49:126–134

Hallenbeck VJ (2012) Use of high-fidelity simulation for staff education/development: A systematic review of the literature. J Nurses Staff Dev 28(6):260–269

Hardy M (1978) Perspectives on nursing theory. Adv Nurs Sci 1(1):37–48

Heggestad AKT, Nortvedt P, Christiansen B, Konow-Lund A (2016) Undergraduate nursing students' ability to empathize: A qualitative study. Nurs Ethics 25(6):786–795

Hughes J, Nicholson H (eds) (2016) Critical perspectives on applied theatre. Cambridge University Press, Cambridge

Hughes J, Kidd J, McNamara C (2011) The usefulness of mess: artistry, improvisation and decomposition in the practice of research in applied theatre. In: Kershaw B, Nicholson H (eds) Research Methods in Theatre and Performance, pp 186–209

Hulkko P, Laakkonen R (2022) Actor education, object animation and care. Theatre, Dance Perform Train 13(2):309–323

Hummelvoll J, Karlsson B, Borg M (2015) Recovery and person-centredness in mental health services: roots of the concepts and implications for practice. Int Pract Dev J 5. Available from: https://www.fons.org/Resources/Documents/Journal/Vol5Suppl/IPDJ_05(suppl)_07.pdf. Accessed 15 Mar 2018

Jackson T (2007) Theatre, education and the making of meanings: art or instrument? Manchester University Press, Manchester

Jackson A, Vine C (eds) (2013) Learning through theatre: the changing face of theatre in education, 3rd edn. Routledge, London

Jacobs AC, van Jaarsveldt DE (2016) 'The character rests heavily within me': drama students as standardized patients in mental health nursing education. J Psychiatr Ment Health Nurs 23(3–4):198–206

Jansen DA, Johnson N, Larson G, Berry C, Brenner GH (2009) Nursing faculty perceptions of obstacles to utilizing manikin-based simulations and proposed solutions. Clin Simul Nurs 5(1):9–16

Jennings M, Deeny P, Tizzard-Kleister K (2020) Acts of care: applied drama, 'sympathetic presence' and person-centred nursing. In: Stuart Fisher A, Thompson J (eds) Performing care: new perspectives on socially engaged performance. Manchester University Press, Manchester, pp 187–203

Johnston C (1998) House of games: making theatre from everyday life. Nick Hern, London

Kirby M (1972) On acting and not-acting. Drama Rev: TDR 16(1):3–15

Kitwood T (1997) Dementia reconsidered: the person comes first. Open University Press, Buckingham

Kolb DA (1984) Experiential learning: experience as the source of learning and development. Prentice-Hall, N.J

Kontos PC, Mitchell G, Mistry B, Ballon B (2010) Using drama to improve person-centred dementia care. Int J Older People Nursing 5(2):159–168

Kooken W, Kerr N (2018) Blending the liberal arts and nursing: creating a portrait for the 21st century. J Prof Nurs 34(1):60–64

Kyle R, Bastow F, Harper-McDonald B, Jeram T, Zahid Z, Nizamuddin M, Mahoney C (2023) Effects of student-led drama on nursing students' attitudes to interprofessional working and nursing advocacy: a pre-test post-test educational intervention study. Nurse Educ Today 123:1–11

Lateef F (2010) Simulation-based learning: just like the real thing. J Emerg Trauma Shock 3(4):348–352

Lawrence J, Wier J (2018) The use of drama within midwifery education to facilitate the understanding of professional behaviour and values. Midwifery 59:59–61

Lazzari C (2011) The use of (silent) mannequins to teach communication skills to medical students: an experimental approach in Italy. Med Teach 33(9):772–772

Leahy R (2002) A model of emotional schemas. Cogn Behav Pract 9:177–190

Lehmann H (2006) Post-dramatic theatre. Routledge, London

Lepp M (2002) Reflections on drama in nursing education in Sweden. Appl Theatr Res 3:1–6

Levett-Jones T, Lapkin S (2014) A systematic review of the effectiveness of simulation debriefing in health professional education. Nurse Educ Today 34:58–63

Loth J, Andersen P, Mitchell P (2015) Acting for health: effective actor preparation for health-care simulations. Appl Theatr Res 3(3):285

Low K (2020) Applied theatre and sexual health communication: apertures of possibility. Palgrave Macmillan, London

Macneill P, Gilmer J, Samarasekera DD, Hoon TC (2014) Actor training for doctors and other healthcare practitioners: a rationale from an actor's perspective. Glob J Arts Educ 4(2):49–55

Macneill P, Gilmer J, Tan CH, Samarasekera DD (2016) Enhancing doctors' and healthcare professionals' patient-care role through actor-training: workshop participants' responses. Ann Acad Med 45(5):205–211

McAllister M, Levett-Jones T, Arthur C, Downer T, Harrison P, Layh J, Harvey T, Reid-Searl K, Calleja P, Lynch K (2013a) Snapshots of simulation: creative strategies used by Australian educators to enhance simulation learning experiences for nursing students. Nurse Educ Pract 13(6):567–572

McAllister M, Reid-Searl K, Davis S (2013b) Who is that masked educator? Deconstructing the teaching and learning processes of an innovative humanistic simulation technique. Nurse Educ Today 33(12):1453–1458

McCance T (2003) Caring in nursing practice: the development of a conceptual framework. Res Theory Nurs Pract 17(2):101–116

McCormack B (2001a) Autonomy and the relationship between nurses and older people. Ageing Soc 21(4):417–446

McCormack B (2001b) Negotiating partnerships with older people: a person centred approach. Ashgate, Aldershot; Burlington, VT

McCormack B, McCance T (2006) Development of a framework for person-centred nursing. J Adv Nurs 56(5):472–479

McCormack B, McCance T (2010) Person-centred nursing: theory and practice. Wiley-Blackwell, Chichester

McCormack B, McCance T (eds) (2016) Person-centred practice in Nursing and Health Care, 2nd edn. Wiley-Blackwell, Chichester

McCormack B, Borg M, Cardiff S, Dewing J, Jacobs G, Janes N, Karlsson B, McCance T, Mekki T, Porock D, Lieshout F, Wilson V (2015) Person-centredness—the 'state' of the art. Int Pract Dev J 5(1):1–15

McCullough M (2012) The art of medicine: bringing drama into medical education. Lancet 379:512–513

McEvoy L, Duffy A (2008) Holistic practice—A concept analysis. Nurse Educ Pract 8(6):412–419

Mermikides A (2020) Performance, medicine and the human. Methuen Drama, London

Middlewick Y, Kettle TJ, Wilson JJ (2012) Curtains up! Using forum theatre to rehearse the art of communication in healthcare education. Nurse Educ Pract 12(3):139–142

Monden KR, Gentry L, Cox TR (2016) Delivering bad news to patients. Bayl Univ Med Cent Proc 29(1):101–102

Moreno J, Moreno Z (1972) Psychodrama: volume 1. Beacon, New York

Neilson SJ, Reeves A (2019) The use of a theatre workshop in developing effective communication in paediatric end of life care. Nurse Educ Pract 36:7–12

Nicholson H (2005) Applied drama: the gift of theatre. Palgrave, Basingstoke

Nicholson N (2011) Theatre, education and performance. Palgrave Macmillan, London

Nicholson H (2017) Affective Labours of cultural participation. In: Harpin A, Nicholson H (eds) Performance and participation: practices, audiences, politics. Palgrave Macmillan, London, pp 105–127

Niessen T, Jacobs G (2015) Curriculum design for person-centredness: mindfulness training within a bachelor course in nursing. International Practice Development Journal. [Online], Available from: https://www.fons.org/Resources/Documents/Journal/Vol5Suppl/IPDJ_05(suppl)_02. pdf. Accessed 6 Mar 2018

Nolan C (2009) Agency and embodiment: performing gestures/producing cultures. Harvard University Press, Harvard

Noonan I, Rafferty AM, Browne J (2016) Creative arts in health professional education and practice: a case study reflection and evaluation of a complex intervention to deliver the culture and care programme at the Florence Nightingale School of Nursing and Midwifery, King's College London. In: Clift S, Camic P (eds) Creative arts, health, and wellbeing: international perspectives on practice, policy, and research. Oxford University Press, Oxford, pp 309–316

Nursing and Midwifery Council (NMC) (2018) Future nurse: Standards for proficiency and practice for registered nurses. NMC. Available from: future-nurse-proficiencies.pdf (nmc.org.uk) Accessed 1 June 2021

O'Connor P, Anderson M (2015) Applied theatre: research, radical departures. Methuen, London

O'Grady A (2017) Introduction: risky aesthetics, critical vulnerabilities, and Edgeplay: tactical performances of the unknown. In: O'Grady A (ed) Risk, participation and performance practice: critical vulnerabilities in a precarious world. Palgrave Macmillan, London, pp 1–29

Patient Client Council (PCC) (2017) Quality report 2016/2017. The Patient Client Council, Belfast. http://www.patientclientcouncil.hscni.net/uploads/research/Q2020_report_2016_17. pdf. Accessed 30 Oct 2018

Perry M, Maffulli N, Willson S, Morrissey D (2011) The effectiveness of arts-based interventions in medical education: a literature review. Med Educ 45:141–148

Plato (2007) Republic. Penguin, London

Randle J, Webb C, Jenkinson T (2003) Making a difference? Teaching communication skills in preregistration nurse education in England. J Res Nurs 8(6):429–438

Reason M, Rowe N (2017) Applied practice: evidence and impact in theatre, music, and art. Bloomsbury, London

Reeves A, Neilson S (2018) 'Don't talk like that: It's not just what you say but how you say it': the process of developing an applied theatre performance to teach undergraduate nursing students communication skills around paediatric end-of-life care. J Appl Arts Health 9(1):99–111

Reeves A, Nyatanga B, Neilsen S (2021) Transforming empathy to empathetic practice amongst nursing and drama students. Res Drama Educ 26(2):1–18

Reid-Searl K, O'Neill B, Dwyer T, Crowley K (2017) Using a procedural puppet to teach paediatric nursing procedures. Clin Simul Nurs 13(1):15–23

Ritzer G (2004) The McDonaldization of society. Sage, London

Schlegel K, Grandjean D, Scherer K (2014) Introducing the Geneva emotion recognition test: an example of Rasch-based test development. Psychol Assess 26(2):666–672

Siassakos D et al (2011) Team communication with patient actors: findings from a multisite simulation study. Simul Healthc 6(3):143–149

Smith M (2015) The practice of applied puppetry: antecedents and tropes. Res Drama Educ 20(4):531–536

Snyder-Young D (2018) No "Bullshit": rigor and evaluation of applied theatre projects. In: Freebody K, Balfour M, Finneran M, Anderson M (eds) Applied theatre: understanding change. Springer, London, pp 81–94

Souza M, Tavares C, Gama L, Passos J (2015) Primer drama—a technical education product. J Res : Fundamental Care Online 7(4):3542–3553

Stanislavski C (1961) Creating a role. Theatre Arts Books, New York

Stanislavski C (1990) An actor's handbook. Methuen, London

Stuart Fisher A, Thompson J (eds) (2020) Performing care: new perspectives on socially engaged performance. Manchester University Press, Manchester

Taylor S, Taylor R (2017) Making power visible: doing theatre-based status work with nursing students. Nurse Educ Pract 26:1–5

Taylor N, Wyres M, Green A, Hennessy-Priest K, Phillips C, Daymond E, Love R, Johnson R, Wright J (2021) Developing and piloting a simulated placement experience for students, in Br J Nurs, 30;13.

The National Archives (TNA): GUK (Records of GOV.UK) (2013) A review of the NHS Hospital Complaints System: putting the patient back into the picture, Available from: https://assets. publishing.service.gov.uk/government/uploads/system/uploads/attachment_data/file/255615/ NHS_complaints_accessible.pdf. Accessed 30 Oct 2018

Thompson J (2015) Towards an aesthetics of care. Res Drama Educ. The Journal of Applied Theatre and Performance 20(4):430–441

Thompson J (2023) Care aesthetics: for artful care and careful art. Routledge, London

Tilbrook A, Dwyer T, Reid-Searl K, Parson J (2017) A review of the literature—the use of interactive puppet simulation in nurses education and children's healthcare. Nurse Educ Pract 22:73–79

Tizzard-Kleister K, Jennings M (2020) "Breath, belief, focus, touch": applied puppetry in simulated role play for person-centred nursing education. Appl Theatr Res 8(1):73–87

Victor J, Ruppert W, Ballasy S (2017) Examining the relationships between clinical judgement, simulation performance, and clinical performance. Nurse Educ 42(5):236–239

Vygotsky LS (1978) Mind in society: development of higher psychological processes. Harvard University Press, Cambridge, Massachusetts

Wasylko Y, Stickley T (2003) Theatre and pedagogy: using drama in mental health nurse education. Nurse Educ Today 23:443–448

Wharram C (2014) Nothing human. Educ Theory 64(5):515–532

Wheeler CA, Mcnelis AM (2014) Nursing student perceptions of a community-based home visit experienced by a role-play simulation. Nurs Educ Perspect 35(4):259–261

White M (2009) Arts development in community health: a social tonic. Radcliffe, Oxford

Williams J, Stickley T (2010) Empathy and nurse education. Nurse Educ Today 30(8):752–755

Willson S (2006) What can the arts bring to medical training? Lancet 368:s15–s16

Willson S, Jaye P (2017) Arts based learning for a circle of care. Lancet 390:642–643

Wilson V, McCance T (2015) Good enough evaluation. Int Pract Dev J 5. Available from: https:// www.fons.org/library/journal/volume5-person-centredness-suppl/article10. Accessed 20 Mar 2018

Wilson C, Bungay H, Munn-Giddings C, Boyce M (2015) Healthcare professionals' perceptions of the value and impact of the arts in healthcare settings: A critical review of the literature. Int J Nurs Stud 56:90–101

Yakhforoshha A, Emami SAH, Mohammadi N, Cheraghi M, Mojtahedzadeh R, Mahmoodi-Bakhtiari B, Shirazi M (2017) Developing an integrated educational simulation model by considering art approach: teaching empathetic communication skills. Eur J Pers Cent Healthc 5(1):154–165

Applying Stanislavski to Nursing Education

3

Applying Stanislavski's Method of Physical Action

This chapter and the next turn towards building a shared conceptual frame for applied drama and person-centred nursing. This chapter will explore Stanislavski's Method of Physical Action (MoPA) and the resonances between this system and person-centred nursing, with particular attention to the topic of education. The next chapter—Chap. 4—builds on this, and on the groundwork laid in Chap. 2, to present a dynamic and cross-discipline framework for understanding how I have approached this interdisciplinary project. It is not comprehensive or exhaustive, and there are certainly other ways to 'do it'. What these chapters present are the elements of crossover that are enlivening and enriching from my perspective as a researcher and practitioner. To start, I wish to critique an approach which has seen some interest in drama and nursing involving an application of Stanislavski's approach, the practice of 'emotion memory' (EM).

A Critique of the Application of Emotion Memory

Stanislavski is widely considered the most influential figure in the most dominant acting style of modern times (Merlin 2014). Stanislavski's life work was focused on creating an approach to acting that could be defined and structured, and that was repeatable, transposable, and rigorous. In many ways, he sought a technical approach to what was a nebulous profession. Stanislavski's intention was for no singular idea or approach to be the focus of his systems and methods, rather he considered the entire process of the whole series of practices as vital. This might be one reason his ideas are less readily used in applied drama practice. Another reason might be that his ideas are already an application. In this case, his system was based on observations of how people act in real life, these observations influenced the creation of techniques for performance and rehearsal to make acting more 'realistic'. As Merlin

© The Author(s), under exclusive license to Springer Nature Switzerland AG 2024
K. Tizzard-Kleister, *Applied Drama and Person-Centred Nursing*,
https://doi.org/10.1007/978-3-031-77208-5_3

(2014) describes, Stanislavski aimed to 'systematise natural (and often unconscious) human responses and organise them into something which could be consciously applied to the artifice of acting' (p. 22). This systematisation became known as 'the system', which at this point included EM. Later, this system was adapted towards what is now known as the MoPA. In the MoPA, Stanislavski consciously moves away from EM as a concept and a practice (Benedetti 1998; Carnicke 2010; Merlin 2014).

Stanislavski has influenced many practitioners, including Lee Strasberg. Strasberg took Stnaislavski's work on, adopting more features from the early version of Stanislavski's 'system' in an approach that relied heavily on the concept of 'affective memory', or EM. Strasberg's adaptation of Stanislavski's 'system' has been influential for acting on screen in what is called 'method acting'. EM is a 'memory which makes you relive the sensations you once felt' to better perform similar emotions in rehearsal and on stage (Stanislavski 1990: p. 55). It is a contentious approach. Some argue it is one of Stanislavski's finest contributions (Strasberg 1987). Others regard it with caution (Adler 2000; Tait 2021). Stanislavski intended the exercise to be an aspect of character development that worked alongside other approaches and suggested that '[t]he broader your emotion memory, the richer your material for inner creativeness' (1990: p. 56). Later, he advises how reliance on personal emotional recall can lead to 'increased power […] over the original feelings experienced' and may make an actor 'faint away when he recalls the memory of it' (Ibid). Many believe that EM allows the actor to get at the 'truth' of a role, by connecting a real memory and associated emotions of the actor to the non-real emotions of the character. However, this is problematised in Stanislavski's later developments which move away from using it. He began to challenge the notion of 'truth' on stage as having to come from a 'real' place. Instead, he considers how '[t]ruth on the stage is not the small external truth […] It is what you can sincerely believe in' (Ibid: p. 23). This shift in thinking shows how it is not necessary for a feeling to be real or truthful to be 'authentically' performed.

I argue that for our purpose of applying drama to nursing education EM is potentially dangerous and mostly unnecessary, particularly when it is used in isolation from the rest of Stanislavski's approaches. There are examples of interventions in healthcare simulation that use this approach in isolation for actors or drama students involved as simulated patients in a healthcare simulation (Walsh and Murphy 2017). There are also examples of EM being taught to nursing students themselves, so they might better perform nursing roles, in what are short-term interventions, with little time to develop a robust understanding of Stanislavski's work (Goodwin and Deady 2013). These projects also tend to focus on empathy. 'Empathy', Tait (2021) explains, 'is considered to arise through thinking and feeling that simulate what another (others) is experiencing' (p. 20). This process of simulating experience is based on assumption and can never truly be the same as what the other is feeling, whilst—like EM—also taking a significant amount of emotional labour to achieve (Hochschild 1983; Smith 1992; Tait 2021). The paradox is doubled, as even when using emotion memory, the emotion brought forth is not the emotion aroused by the original event but the emotion aroused at the *memory* of the event.

As McCormack and McCance (2010) suggest regarding PCN, a nurse can be ill-served by continually drawing on personal experience and emotional reserves, which often reduces their ability to cope and leaves little to offer up to patients, family members, colleagues, and anyone else in their care. I would add that this also leaves little for the nurse as a person regarding their own life. This is a significant reason for my adopting McCormack and McCance's (2010) term sympathetic presence over empathy in this study. This deeply resonates with the choice of using EM or not in applied contexts, where empathy relates more closely to EM and sympathetic presence relates to the later developed MoPA without EM as a practice. As Tait (2021) describes, excluding EM and using the MoPA shows how '[a]n idea of an emotion can determine how intention is acted, and in strategies that use verbs for intention with the emotions expressed as adverbs' (p. 51). In a sense, this moves us beyond the need to feel emotion for that emotion to be expressed or understood. Furthermore, there is a suggestion in this reading of the MoPA that emotions are secondary to action, more precisely that emotion emerges from action rather than the opposite. Crudely—in the frame of actor training and performance—this suggests that one does not throw a chair because one may be angry, rather the action of throwing a chair might denote and express the existence of anger. Perhaps more pleasantly, one does not kiss someone because one loves them, rather it is the kiss that *expresses* that love.[1] In a double step, according to the MoPA, an action also arouses emotion. For example, it may be the act of a kiss evokes feelings of love. The consequence of applying this to nursing is that it may remove the assumed need to feel the pain—or indeed any other feeling—of others to care effectively for them. Rather, it is in our actions that care is realised. Importantly, care is not 'an act', it is within an act, and it is 'active'. How this avoids 'pretence' or being 'demonstrational' rather than 'authentic' is a contentious point.

As Merlin (2001) explains, Stanislavski transferred his 'attention from inner emotion to on-stage action' to avoid 'demonstrational acting' where emotions are demonstrated rather than evoked or simulated (p. 16, p. 15). This avoids the potential of re-traumatisation when accessing emotional memories to aid performance (Baim 2017). Meanwhile, this also provides methods to physicalise emotions through easily performed and safely accessed actions. This positions acting more towards a skill-based approach, where one might learn and develop skills through

---

[1] There are of course contradicting arguments to this point, including - keeping with our example - love that plays out without as visible an act as an embrace or a kiss. Where is the action in love that does not involve words or touch? Does love require an act to be realised? And of course, the often-used dramatic trope of unrequited love - can this be love if it is not reciprocated, accepted, or even acted upon at all? These are worthwhile arguments to explore, though all miss the subtlety and potentiality of an action. An act (or action) can be a thought, a glimpse, or a sense within a fleeting moment. Visible acts, such as a kiss, are simply more obvious and often less encumbered with context and interpretation. An act, or action, at a fairly fundamental point, is as simple as a thought, and so originates from the very kernel of an intent towards another person. It is this that characterises and expresses an emotion. Actions are perhaps the most crucial aspect of the MoPA which has influenced my work and will be explored later in the chapter along with other resonant approaches. Bordering on the *cliché*, it is true that actions speak louder than words.

practice. The main thesis of Stanislavski's MoPA can be said to be 'if the performer actively did something and imaginatively committed to what he or she was doing, appropriate emotions would arise accordingly' (Merlin 2001: p. 16). Merlin (2014: p. 26–7) suggests that many practitioners focus on Stanislavski's psychological approaches—seen in *An Actor Prepares* (Stanislavski 2013a)—rather than his approach to the physical work of an actor—seen in *Creating a Role* (Stanislavski 2013b). Merlin (2001) advocates for a 'psycho-physical' approach by bringing the two fragments of Stanislavski's work together into a 'toolkit' (Merlin 2014). As Stanislavski remarks, 'in each physical act there is an inner psychological motive which impels physical action, as in every psychological inner action there is also physical action, which expresses its psychic nature' (1990: p. 159). This contradicts Tait's (2021) assertion that '[d]rama communicates the emotions through words and languages' (p. 5). Instead, I contend it is more often through sensation and action that feelings and emotions are best expressed. For example, I may say the words 'I love you', but convey little of what we might identify as love. What is often questioned is whether this is authentic or not. Concern over authenticity in these ways and others is interestingly shared with nursing.

This conceptual framing offers an alternative understanding of authenticity which is easier for people to access and maintain through performativity and sympathetic presence using Stanislavski's MoPA as an applied framework. I argue that authenticity need not be found in a sense of 'shared experience' or 'true emotion'. Here authenticity stands in for empathy. For some, EM is a useful way to approach these 'truly felt' emotions through one's personal experience and a way to empathise with 'imagined others'. The issue arises when EM is suggested as a technique to use in performance, rather than in rehearsal. When you are asked to engage more authentically through empathetic terms, you are being asked to give more of yourself over to 'really' connecting, to feeling what others feel directly within yourself. Through sympathetic presence, however, being authentic means knowing yourself, knowing you are different from others, recognising how others feel through attending to the cues they give you and the relation this has to your feelings, and then bringing this knowledge and insight with you in your interactions.

To summarise my critique of EM as an approach for actor training and as a technique to be applied in working in drama and nursing contexts, it erroneously focuses on an internalised performance of a felt authenticity which is analogous to the process of empathy. In short, it asks us to 'use ourselves' to understand others and I believe this is impossible. In comparison, sympathetic presence and the MoPA cultivate performativity which finds authenticity and understanding not within one person, but in reciprocal interaction and action felt, sensed, and translated between people. Moreover, many drama approaches are well-positioned to promote the performativity of sympathetic presence. The next section looks towards Stanislavski's MoPA for specific practices and concepts to this end.

A Closer Look at Four Key Techniques

The potential to apply Stanislavski's techniques beyond the stage is mostly untapped by applied drama scholars and practitioners, let alone those interested in working in health. Below is an overview and description of resonant aspects of Stanislavski's approaches to actor training and suggestions on how they might be applied to nursing education and the contexts of this study. This section is influenced by, and extends, the work of Jennings et al. (2020). It is also a close reading of Stanislavski's *An Actor's Handbook* (1990) applied to nursing education. *An Actor's Handbook* is a bringing together of Stanislavski's collated works in a succinct and accessible text. This text is the main source for this section, but it is worth remembering that this text is made up of extracts from the majority of Stanislavski's published works along with Stanislavski's commentary on them—and so the ideas will be present in other texts. The decision to use this singular text instead of drawing from each publication individually reflects Stanislavski's desire to bring his ideas together. The benefit of this is in how when talking about, say, the concept of actions this one text pulls together all of Stanislavski's sources to articulate an overarching view of the concept in his own words. This therefore includes Stanislavski's hindsight and experience with ideas which in earlier texts might be relatively new and under-explored.

Actions

Stanislavski describes that though 'everything that happens on the stage has a definite purpose' these 'actions' do not only refer to overt physical activity, suggesting that '[y]ou may sit without motion and at the same time be in full action' (Stanislavski 1990: p. 8). In *An Actor's Handbook* (1990), he describes three main ways actions are considered in his actor training approach; as 'physical actions'; as actions which contribute to 'the physical life of a role'; and as actions which form a pattern informing a character (Ibid: p. 8).

Physical actions are simply that, something one physically does. These actions might be small but 'acquire an enormous inner meaning' and often lead an actor—and at times an audience—to a 'true objective' (Ibid). Meanwhile, these physical actions ensure that one avoids forcing emotions to the surface, instead accessing emotional states which are 'natural, intuitive and complete' through performing actions (Ibid). For Stanislavski, the effectiveness—in terms of realism—of physical action on stage is reliant on the actor having 'faith in their reality' (Ibid). He considered this faith vital for the actor to access their 'inner creative state' (Ibid).

I argue that this might be the case for this form of acting, which seeks to present naturalism on stage, but inner creative states as a wider term can also be accessed through disbelief. This means that creating a compelling and 'authentic' performance can both acknowledge the non-reality of performance and commit to it anyway. I do not mean to suggest that Stanislavski reduces the notion of an actor's creativity to rely on faith in the actions they play, but that this feature is specifically related to an acting context based on presenting naturalistic realism on stage. As such it would be a difficult concept to include when placing Stanislavski's techniques outside of their original context. For example, it might be too far a step to ask nursing students to fully 'commit' to their faith in their actions after a short introduction to Stanislavski's ideas. Particularly when this is not to produce a 'performance', but for developing a robust ability to be 'performative'. It would be unethical to teach this approach as a way for nursing students to perform emotions (or to put it bluntly, to 'fake it'), instead, it is a pathway to develop skills in performativity of emotional interaction. Seen in this way, applying the MoPA and the concept of actions in particular offers nursing students a pathway to explore different actions and ways to interact, developing their communicative potential without prescribing one particular way of communication as a one-size-fits-all approach. As such, rather than encourage nursing students to perform 'physical actions' with absolute belief, it may be more suitable to direct them to perform actions 'as if' this situation was a real one whilst acknowledging that this is not real. This is an important facet of applying Stanislavski's MoPA, as it moves away from performing naturalistic actions at that moment. Instead, actions are a way to practice, develop, and rehearse a future naturalism for that person in their real life. This also acknowledges that this is practising for a future that is not set. Unlike in acting, interactions in nursing care are not scripted. The uncertainty of how an interaction may play out may be a significant cause of anxiety for many students (the notion of uncertainty creating anxiety in nursing care will be explored more in the next chapter), and practising how you might interact may increase your confidence for future interactions.

Actions also help to create a life-like role. Stanislavski argues that '[t]he spirit cannot but respond to the actions of the body', and so actions inherently contribute to the creation of a role by giving physical and spiritual life to a role (Ibid: p. 9). This allows the actor to focus less on questions like 'what might this character do' and instead to develop an ability to allow this to occur spontaneously, by intuitively constructing and interpreting the 'spirit' of a role through performing and embodying actions. This might be the most resonant aspect of the concept of 'actions' in developing the interactivity of a nursing student. Just as this frees the actor from the constraints of cognitively wrestling with an unsolvable conundrum of what another person is truly thinking, feeling, and doing, it might also do the same for the nursing students. By focusing on physical action, 'analysis'—the intellectual and emotional understanding of a role or a person—'naturally and imperceptibly goes on inside of us' (Ibid: p. 20). It is an embodied exploration, an embodied knowing (Nolan 2009).

From a standpoint of acting, this allows a person to act in a way that may contradict what they perceive as their personhood. For example, the concept of actions might help a person who considers themselves kind, introverted, and thoughtful to perform actions that characterise them as ruthless, extrovert, and callous. More dramatically, it can help a pacifist perform the role of a murderer in a play. Clearly, this is not the best aim when applying these ideas to nursing. A better aim would be for a person who feels unable to communicate in a certain way to find a path to doing so. For example, understanding how to perform a variety of actions may offer someone who thinks of themselves as shy to take action to speak up or for someone who habitually speaks too often to take more listening actions. Considered in this way, one may be encouraged to see beyond how one perceives oneself as a limiting and limited agent in the world. Rather we can begin to realise the huge untapped potential to interact with others through consciously performed actions. This moves physical action beyond a simple mimetic representation, a record of events represented exactly 'as they happened', but as a point in the process of the life of that other person. As such, an action characterises a person. Importantly, 'the point of physical actions lies not in themselves as such but in what they evoke' (Stanislavski 1990: p. 9). This might be somewhat revelatory for nursing students, who to this point may have been taught that caring for their patients relies more on performing specific technical procedures efficiently. Considering the evocation of these actions through Stanislavskian actor training might bring to light what these actions 'do' to others beyond the obvious and into the realms of the 'psycho-physical' (Merlin 2001, 2014).

Lastly, a person's pattern of actions—in this case specifically in a play text—can 'map out' the plot of the play as well as 'engender [...] the life of a human spirit in a role' (Stanislavski 1990: p. 10). Again, I argue that when applying this notion, it must be adapted to make sense in a real-life contextual environment beyond the confines of a play text designed for performance. However, the technique still 'works' when looking at a situation as an abstract one. For instance, examining the actions and patterns of actions in a short improvised interaction between a person playing the role of a nurse and another playing the role of a patient might help reveal things about each person, as well as help to find better ways of interacting. This has the potential to serve beyond education as an approach to analysing interactions in care environments. For Stanislavski mapping out these actions 'is the initial step of merging with and living your part' (Ibid). Although a nurse's role is not scripted or 'acted out', this process might give nursing students insight into how they might 'live their part' as a nurse, as well as how others live their own 'parts' beyond the locus of the nurse's control and perception. This is reflected in how Stanislavski views 'character' not as just external, but as somewhat internal; where the actor does not 'lose his own individuality and his personality' but instead finds it within each role (Ibid: p. 32). Similarly, the nurses need not 'put on' a character based on inauthenticity and fiction, but to find a way to perform a role with their personality 'put into' it. Though I agree with Stanislavski's approach that internalises the psychology of character within us, I also argue that this is concretised through interactions with others, often in surprising ways. We may think we are a caring person, perhaps we believe ourselves to be a good listener as part of our psychological make-up. Even to the point that we feel this defines our 'character'. However, it is the action of 'listening' that dramatically realises (Goffman 1990) this internalised trait, as one that is external, inter-relational, and thereby authentic. It is the action *behind* the kiss that actualises the love, not the love that actualises the kiss.[2]

---

[2]One thing I wish to mention about actions is the notion of 'negative' and 'positive' actions or rather ones people find more or less comfortable to use and have used on them. I often use the

Objectives

Stanislavski discusses how 'objectives' can be identified within a play text and help the actor to see how each part of their performance contains 'a creative objective' (Stanislavski 1990: p. 103). These objectives are things characters want to achieve and much of a performance's interest lies in how a character might overcome the barriers they face in achieving these objectives. Exploring 'objectives' is a way to develop a character and identify their desires, whilst it can help an actor remain true to the character during a performance. This is particularly so for improvisation, where there are fewer structural aids for the actor to maintain this character. For instance, when improvising a character who wants to leave a room without raising concern from any of the other characters, every 'action' an actor performs in character is done to achieve this. They might make an excuse—such as needing to visit the lavatory—to exit without arousing suspicion. These objectives are part of the subconscious of the character which must be consciously identified, explored, and understood by the actor to create the feeling of subconsciousness, spontaneity, and subsequently a sense of reality—or fidelity—in the character's actions. As Stanislavski states, a 'physical objective will contain something of a psychological objective', more specifically the actualisation of a physical objective creates a suitable 'psychological state' (Ibid). At the same time, he warns of 'purely [...] motor [objectives] which [...] lead to mechanical performance' (Ibid: p. 104). As such, an 'objective' must be relevant and must be achievable, but not so simple or contrived that it makes the character's actions in achieving them uninteresting. These objectives must also be 'truthful so that you yourself, the actors playing with you and your audience, can believe in their clear-cut [purpose]' (Ibid: p. 103–4).

The notion of identifying an 'objective' within an interaction offers an approach for nursing students to better understand both their desires and needs, and the desires and needs of others. Objectives are also a way for nursing students to consider interactions from an abstract analytical standpoint, with clear and practical terminology for changing the interaction. What the notion of objectives offers us is an insight into our own goals and a greater focus and engagement with the goals of others. In dramatic storytelling, the objectives of different characters often clash to create compelling dramatic situations. Conversely, when developing communication skills for nursing the aim should be to increase awareness of one's objectives and the objectives of others, to avoid clashes and to aim towards mutuality. Exploring objectives in SRP offers nursing students a structured and responsive approach to communicating clearly and in a person-centred way. In short, objectives offer a communicative strategy that is responsive rather than prescriptive. Where some approaches to communication skills suggest specific techniques—like eye contact, using first names, being at the same level as the other person, and so on—focusing

---

metaphor of a painter's palette to explain that actions in an interaction are like colours in a painting. When we limit the amount of colours we use, it is harder to paint a full picture. Likewise with actions, if we limit ourselves to habitual actions, we limit our potentiality to interact with depth and effectiveness.

on what your objective is as well as trying to discern the objectives of others, leads one to an improvisational approach to person-centred communication skills. The 'actions' or techniques one performs, should all contribute to achieving your and others' objectives. For example, if my objective is to calm someone irritated, I align the actions I perform to this end. I may speak calmly, soften my body language, acknowledge the other person's frustrations, and so on, but these techniques arise from a skilled interpretation of what I want to achieve and performing actions that recognise this. Meanwhile, I must involve a sympathetic presence which helps me recognise how I am feeling and how the other person is feeling, helping me to identify the objective of the other person as (often) distinct from my own.

Helping others to achieve their objective is often an excellent way to help one achieve your objective. For example, the other person may be irritated, and they may have an unconscious objective to get answers to their questions. The longer one is unaware of the other person's objective, the longer it will take to achieve your objective of calming them. In this example, until they have the answers they want, they are far less likely to be calm, whilst any distraction from their objective will serve the opposite purpose and continue or intensify their irritation.[3] Of course, this is not entirely generalisable, every situation is contextual (a feature addressed in a later section on 'given circumstances') and we can always only ever assume what someone else's objective truly is. One useful strategy may be to clearly state your objective and to directly ask what the other person's objective is. This hopefully avoids too much assumption, and any confusion around intent and how that intent is perceived. For example, you may say 'I need you to calm down, but I understand that there is something you need first, can you tell me what it is you need so I can help?'[4]

This moves communication away from intent from one perspective, to intent between both perspectives. It may not be your intent to irritate someone else, but your actions may have the unintended consequence of doing so. Focusing on objectives and developing interactive skill sets offer an approach to communication that aligns your actions with your intentions, and recognising that the other person has their perspective on that action based on their intent and objective. This approach is not a set of scripted techniques. It requires practice to develop it as a skill. Experienced nurses have had time to do just that and can demonstrate incredible

---

[3] I hope this example is universal enough. If it helps, think of a time you had to call an official department with an issue you want to resolve. How often has the person on the other end of the call not tried to help you achieve your objective, but passed you to other departments, asked for information you have already supplied, tried to dismiss you, and so on? It is, understandably, irritating. I hope you have had the opposite experience as well, where the person you have called has sympathetically recognised your objective (and your irritation!) and has directly helped you to achieve it whilst keeping you reassured.

[4] To note, I am a firm believer in the importance of subtext, so for me, it is not necessarily the words you say that carry the most importance and meaning, but how you say them. In this example, stating your objective, and asking the other to state theirs is at its core a listening action, and should be performed as such. Just stating the words 'I need x, what do you need?' isn't enough, one needs to perform actions such as listening, acknowledging, respecting, and so on.

skill at understanding their own and other's objectives and have developed a variety of techniques to help achieve both their own and other people's objectives. I argue that exploring the MoPA and the concept of objectives makes this a purposeful and conscious approach to person-centred communication that can be taught and practiced. I argue that exploring this approach may give a stepping stone between an abstract experience (like 'theory' in university) and real experience (like experience on practice placements). Similar to other acting methods, commitment to objectives enhances the reality and distinctiveness of a performance. The perceived irony of Stanislavski's approach to acting is in how it uses 'true' impulses to contribute to a 'fictional' performance. As Staislavski states:

> To play truly means to be right, logical, coherent, to think, strive, feel and act in unison with your role. If you take all these internal processes, and adapt them to your spiritual and physical life of the person you are representing, we call that living the part. To play truly, you must follow the course of right objectives, like posts to guide you across a tireless plain. (*Ibid*: p.149-50)

Given Circumstances

Stanislavski succinctly defines 'given circumstances' as 'all the circumstances that are given to an actor to take into account as he creates his role' (Ibid: p. 67). Though this is simple in conception, it soon adds increasing layers of complexity to a role through introducing more circumstances to a situation. For Stanislavski, this process helps an actor in the development and exploration of their role—and more so of one's understanding of that role as another person. Given circumstances can be defined as the context that the 'character' finds themselves within. In our application, given circumstances can offer a way for the abstract concepts of actor training to come to life for nursing students. Applying interesting, relevant, and difficult circumstances to the simulated encounters and role plays tasks nursing students to imaginatively and physically navigate a huge variety of events. I argue that it is at this point at which many examples of drama applied to nursing start. Most examples of projects which apply drama to nursing forgo the preparation and skills-based elements of the dramatic approach. Instead, they jump immediately into using drama as a method to explore a given circumstance in a different way for nursing students. This may include watching or taking part in a 'dramatised' event with particular circumstances. What is missing are the preparations, techniques, and processes that help us to better understand, engage in, and change these scenarios, such as actions and objectives.

Stanislavski remarks that the 'given circumstances' must be preceded by belief, more specifically with the actor conducting 'the Magic If', where the actor imagines what they might do if they were in a similar situation. For this applied context, I argue that applying these given circumstances to the nursing students is the exact moment at which they are invited to engage with 'the Magic If'. However, where Stanislavski might suggest that this is compulsory for the actor to have already done and indeed accepted, I argue that for the nursing students, this might not be the case.

This application intends to encourage the students to actively ask the question 'What would I do', but in this circumstance, it is alongside the application of context—of the 'given circumstances'. 'The Magic If' will see more attention in Chap. 4, contributing to the shared conceptual framing of this work.

In practice, an awareness of given circumstances gives life to role play, simulation, or improvisation. For example, a scene may be explored where a nurse is trying to calm a patient who is looking for answers. Both may be performing relevant and realistic actions, and committing to achieving their objectives. However, if a given circumstance is added then the context of the scene changes, it adds a new 'what if' to the scenario. For instance, what if the nurse has been working for 12 hours, is sore in their whole body, has a headache, and is emotionally drained? Or what if the patient needs answers to their questions because they have been called to the hospital because their loved one has had a serious accident, and they need to find them— under it all they are terrified that they may never see their loved one again unless they get answers right now. What if the two are estranged ex-lovers? What if they do not speak the same language? What if the nurse has another critically ill patient they must return to as soon as they can? What if the nurse has just argued with a colleague? What if the patient has been waiting to be seen for 5 hours?

Hopefully, it is clear that when using given circumstances in a rehearsal process we can creatively explore interactions, and demonstrate how the scenario might drastically change if the given circumstances are changed. What this approach also leads to is an awareness of the context in a real-life situation. It might give us an insight that a person who appears angry, is performing threatening actions, and has an objective to get answers as quickly as possible, might be deeply fearful of losing their loved one, and needs reassurance and support not to be simply labelled 'an angry person'. This may contradict the earlier assertion that actions characterise us, but in this case, it is not as simple as the action 'to threaten' makes one a threatening person. Rather, the action 'to threaten' characterises their behaviour at that moment in time. Undeniably, they are a threatening person at that moment, however, this should not be considered who they always are, as this leads to an assumption of essentialism for their character as *always* threatening. They are not 'Miss Johnson', they are 'that angry lady'. In this, we easily miss the context and given circumstance that has led to this behaviour. We may miss other parts of them, as we assume anger is the culprit for their behaviour, rather than the circumstance. I am steadfast in my contention that the vast majority of people do not act on their emotions alone, rather they embody and express emotions as a consequence of the circumstances they find themselves in. Meanwhile, we are all guilty of focusing more on the emotions of others (and ourselves) rather than the circumstances that generate those emotions for that person, or indeed for ourselves. Engaging with the given circumstance of a situation helps us to see persons more holistically, and in a more person-centred way. We see 'them'. We see them as a multiplicity, not as a reduced, singular, aspect.

Attention

Developing an actor's ability to pay attention is a key aspect of Stanislavski's approach, particularly in paying attention to sensations. In the same way that being consciously aware of a character's 'objectives' helps the actor to create what appears to be a subconscious performance of that role, conscious attention helps to bring a natural subconscious attentiveness to a role. Stanislavski describes five main aspects to consider regarding attention: concentration; sensory concentration; imaginary objects; physical attention; and creative material.

For Stanislavski, attention as concentration must be focused and spatially located for the actor, it must be 'on the stage and the stage alone' (Ibid: p. 24). For our application to nursing education, the stage is not important, but the localisation of concentration becomes vital. Stanislavski calls this a 'circle of attention'. For instance, are you concentrating on a singular person? On a person and family member? A person and the observation equipment? For nursing students, concentration should be consciously identified to understand where one's concentration is and to recognise where it is most needed. For example, I have often observed role plays where nursing students more readily interact with family members who are more able to talk than the patient who may be limited in their verbal capacity. Often the patient feels ignored. Applying Stanislavski's concept of attention as a practice can offer a way where both the patient and family members are given suitable attention. As Stanislavski suggests, when one pays attention to something one's 'desire to do something with it' is increased, which in turn 'intensifies your observation of it' (Ibid). The implication is that the more attention we pay to a patient, the more we wish to interact with them. Perhaps when a patient is the concentrated point of attention for the student nurses, they more readily centralise that person to their practice.

Next, Stanislavski highlights the potential of 'sensory attention'. With concentration as a first step, it is then necessary to engage with what one pays attention to with more than mechanical attention as simply an intensity of focus. Instead one 'must learn to transfigure an object from something which is coldly reasoned or intellectual in quality into something which is warmly felt' (Ibid: p. 25). This can be likened to an awareness of what the centre of your attention is doing to you on the level of sensation. It is listening to one's feelings and using one's senses to flesh out the aspects of what is being attended to. Deeply intertwined with this need to engage sensations with what one pays attention to are 'imaginary objects', which 'centres on things we see, hear and touch and feel in imaginary circumstances' (Ibid). Harnessing sensations and imagination are vital for an actor to develop and perform a life-like role. Applying these ideas might develop a nursing student's ability to engage with what they pay attention to in a sensuous and holistic way. Imagination and attentiveness are undervalued qualities in nursing education. Through conscious attention to objects in an imaginative sense, nursing students may cultivate new ways of seeing, practising, and being, that would have otherwise been ignored. Here I argue imagination offers a counter to mechanisation, as well as a pathway to creative problem-solving.

Lastly, Stanislavski describes how attention to one's 'physical' aspects draws attention to one's tensions and existence, whilst highlighting the need to engage with 'creative material' so that one's ability to pay attention does not become just 'a scientific technique' (Ibid: p. 26, 27). Crucial here is the mixture and balance of both intellectual work and creative expression. For actors to attend to themselves and others effectively they must complete 'an immense amount of work' before drawing on 'the living emotional material' so they may 'stimulate [their] subconscious selves' (Ibid: p. 26). This is remarkably similar to the nurse, who also must complete huge amounts of this 'work' before interacting with their patients, family members, and often colleagues, especially when they first meet others. Through paying 'physical' attention a nursing student might better develop skills in observation, and an ability to interpret features in others which give rich information on their lives and personhood in that given moment.

This technique of attention created for actors is not entirely technical nor entirely sensory, it is a marriage of both. This combination may deeply enhance a nursing student's ability to recognise features in others. Though 'many invisible, spiritual experiences are reflected in our facial expression', Stanislavski reminds us that 'people do not often open the doors of their souls' (Ibid). As a result, we should be wary of assumptions, and be constantly mindful that what we discern in the physicality of others is always our interpretation, not necessarily 'the truth'. What we feel we know about what others are feeling and thinking is not—and perhaps can never be—objective truth. We can certainly get close to it but there will, it seems, always be a gap. However, by paying close attention to others and building strong relationships with them we are at least trying to get closer to understanding their feelings and experiences through recognising features of how they present themselves. Moreover, we must be keenly and constantly aware that paying deep attention to others in this way is taxing, laborious, and often intense. However, it is also often rewarding, invigorating, life-sustaining, and deeply human. Continuing the previous thread, attentiveness is perhaps the exact opposite of a mechanical and technical task-based approach to healthcare work.

Applying these ideas to nursing students may help to enhance their ability to engage with others on an emotional level. It may help them to pay attention to themselves and their physical presence and to pay attention to the features and aspects of others with more finesse. As such, they may be less inclined to ignore the creative and sensuous aspects of their work. As Stanislavski eloquently puts it, '[d]o not be a cold observer of another's life, but let [your study] raise your own creative temperature' (Ibid: p. 27). This speaks to the importance of what one might learn using one's attention and the fullness of feeling one engages in the creative process of being with and paying attention to others. I feel strongly that this is an area of strength for PCN. This, along with the other elements of Stanislavski's MoPA explored earlier, lights an intriguing pathway for nursing education to cultivate creative skills in interactivity, and a person-centred care practice that avoids mechanism and embraces a person-centred humanism.

For Stanislavski, this was intended for actors in their training and rehearsal, and the 'other' in question is often an abstract other, a character in a play for example.

When applied to person-centred nursing this other is never abstracted, but always personal, embodied, present. If anything, this makes the skill of attention even more important for nurses than for actors. Simply, for nurses the people they attend to are often in contexts where they are 'at risk', 'in danger', or 'vulnerable'. It is a nurse's priority and responsibility that these persons do not come to harm. This 'attentiveness', then, is a key element of care, as Tronto's model of care ethics reminds us, positing attentiveness as a necessity for care delivery (2013: p. 34). As Jennings et al. (2020) state, '[t]he cultivation of conscious attentiveness can help carers to recognise and clarify their intentions (both conscious and subconscious) and the consequences of their actions within the caring relationship' (p. 194). Before this skill can flourish, there are some lingering questions to address, such as those posed by the entangling of risk, danger, uncertainty, harm, and vulnerability in healthcare. The pertinent question for our context is how to encourage risk-taking so that one can be attentive and, as Stanislavski puts it, raise one's 'creative temperature' (Stanislavski 1990: p. 27), without unconscious distraction or anxiety. This is how the next chapter will open, and then progress to develop a conceptual frame built through the coming together of concepts explored in the preceding chapters.

References

Adler S (2000) The art of acting. Applause, New York

Baim C (2017) The drama spiral: a decision making model for safe, ethical, and flexible practice when incorporating personal stories in applied theatre and performance. In: O'Grady A (ed) Risk, participation, and performance practice: critical vulnerabilities in a precarious world. Palgrave Macmillan, London, pp 79–109

Benedetti J (1998) Stanislavski and the actor. Methuen Drama, London

Carnicke SM (2010) Stanislavsky's system: pathways for the actor. In: Hodge A (ed) Actor training. Routledge, Abingdon, pp 28–53

Goffman E (1990) The presentation of self in everyday life. Penguin, London

Goodwin J, Deady R (2013) The art of mental health practice: the role of Drama in developing empathy. Perspect Psychiatr Care 49:126–134

Hochschild AR (1983) The managed heart. University of California Press, Berkeley

Jennings M, Deeny P, Tizzard-Kleister K (2020) Acts of care: applied drama, 'sympathetic presence' and person-centred nursing. In: Stuart Fisher A, Thompson J (eds) Performing care: new perspectives on socially engaged performance. Manchester University Press, Manchester, pp 187–203

McCormack B, McCance T (2010) Person-centred nursing: theory and practice. Wiley-Blackwell, Chichester

Merlin B (2001) Beyond Stanislavski: the psycho-physical approach to actor training. Routledge, New York

Merlin B (2014) The complete Stanislavski toolkit. Nick Hern, New York

Nolan C (2009) Agency and embodiment: performing gestures/producing cultures. Harvard University Press, Harvard

Smith P (1992) The emotional labour of nursing: its impact on interpersonal relations, management and educational environments. Palgrave, Basingstoke

Stanislavski C (1990) An actor's handbook. Methuen, London

Stanislavski C (2013a) An actor prepares. Bloomsbury, London

Stanislavski C (2013b) Creating a role. Bloomsbury, London

Strasberg L (1987) A dream of passion: the development of the method. Little, Brown & Co, Boston
Tait P (2021) Theory for theatre studies: emotion. Methuen drama, London
Tronto J (2013) Caring democracy: markets, equality, and justice. New York University Press, New York
Walsh IK, Murphy P (2017) Healtheatre: drama and medicine in concert. Healthcare 5:3

Building a Shared Conceptual Frame

4

Introduction

This chapter will summarise the first part of this book by drawing the topics and ideas together to form a shared conceptual framing for the conjunction of applied drama and person-centred nursing. This chapter represents an approach to interdisciplinarity where disciplines meet as an application of one to the other and as a mutual exchange at a conceptual level. I argue this is far from just a speculative exercise, rather it is a major benefit of interdisciplinary practice, where new and emerging concepts and approaches are reached through a process of metaphorical translation across disciplines. As mentioned earlier, this is not an exhaustive or all-encompassing framework, nor it is not a set of guidelines or principles. It is an accumulation of experience and analysis on the topics and how they intersect, lighting a path for ways to bring the disciplines together and create new approaches for both. One resonant starting point is the concept of risk.

Person-Centred Nursing and Cultural Aversion to Risk

Although taking certain risks is identified as a key factor in training practitioners (Titchen et al. 2017), a cultural aversion to risk is still a significant barrier for this to be implemented into nursing education (Dingwall et al. 2017). As Jennings et al (2020) state '[p]ractitioners are required to be open in their communication with those they care for and are often required to advocate on their behalf', however, 'this is not possible until a practitioner first 'knows themselves" and is comfortable with their vulnerabilities' (p. 202). What is less addressed is the difficulty with approaching vulnerabilities in cultures which have transferred the notion of risk aversion from areas such as germ theory into emotional risk-taking. In many respects, this is due to the pervasiveness of the biomedical model of health. This section does not seek to critique the biomedical model of health, instead, I hope to critique the effect

© The Author(s), under exclusive license to Springer Nature Switzerland AG 2024
K. Tizzard-Kleister, *Applied Drama and Person-Centred Nursing*, https://doi.org/10.1007/978-3-031-77208-5_4

of an overreliance on this model, and how when applied to all healthcare all of the time, the biomedical model promotes a risk aversion that is often insurmountable for person-centred practice to challenge the ill effects of mechanisation and task-based care. This section will attempt to disentangle the concept of risk with the concepts of danger, uncertainty, and vulnerability from their housing in a purely biomedical frame. Instead, I will present a person-centred point of view on these terms aided by the perspective of performance studies. I do not wish to suggest that the biomedical view of these terms be disregarded but hope to present an argument for a balance between this and a person-centred view.

Below is a short excerpt from my journal detailing an SRP session I attended from the UU module 'The Safe and Effective Nurse' as part of the beginning stages of my doctoral study. This experience gave me a first-hand experience of how risk creates a barrier for PCN. This experience led me to explore ideas of risk within PCN more closely. This extract will be used as an example throughout this section. I hope it illustrates the need to combine a biomedical approach with a person-centred one.

A Nursing lecturer and I were watching a group practice their SRP the week before their assessment. We were offering feedback as they showed us what they had developed. The group was doing well and each group member was responding to both my colleague's directions on improving their technical nursing skills as well as my advice on improving their interactions with each other and their simulated patient (performed by a medical mannequin). They had determined that their simulated patient - Annie - had a possible infection, and this should be checked, and samples taken. The student who seemed to be taking the lead mentioned to the tutor that she was now going to create a 'sterile field' before observing the wound site for possible infection and taking samples. The tutor nodded approvingly. I was intrigued, I hadn't come across this term or procedure and was impressed with their proactiveness in adding this into the role-play. This procedure was not part of the stated expectations of the role-play, the group took the initiative to include it. What happened next was mesmerising. Under a cloak of intense silence and focus the lead student purposefully began to gather together the things she needed. Each motion began to take on more and more importance as a sterile field was created and sustained. Slowly and carefully gloves, aprons, plastic sheeting, and various pieces of equipment were unwrapped. With each new item unwrapped the group's movements began to flow with increased care and attention, as they worked as a group to ensure each item remained perfectly sterile. The lead student would carefully tear the corners of packets, gently pull the item out, unfold it and almost lovingly place it down onto a sterile plastic sheet on a trolley at the patient's bedside. Meanwhile, the rest of the group buzzed around her, removing used parts as rubbish, clearing pathways, and supporting her in her motions. Once every item was in place, they began to simulate observation and sampling. I was astonished at the attention paid to each step in this five-minute process. It was choreography and it was nothing short of beautiful.

The Nursing lecturer sang the group's praises, remarking that the sterile field was created perfectly. I was somewhat awed, which only increased as the lecturer commented in detail on the technical procedure, using words like 'aseptic technique' and 'surgical scrub', which made little sense to me. After offering her thoughts, my colleague asked me if I had any comments for the group. Initially, I was speechless. After thinking for a second, something struck me. Firstly, I praised the group, not just for including the creation of a sterile field, but for simulating it so effectively. I also noted that it was a privilege to watch, and the students clearly showed they absolutely knew what they were doing with this technical skill. Then I asked; in the five minutes or so it took to enact this task, did Annie become more scared, or less? They initially didn't know how to answer, before one of them quickly said, 'Of course less scared, she said yes to it happening and she knows she is being cared for'. I agreed that their patient had consented, but after this, Annie had been completely ignored whilst the team set up the sterile field, so how did they know the patient was or was not scared? Or felt cared for? Silence. I noted that the patient would have no clue as to the importance of what the nurses were doing, or how it was providing care for them and in paying so much attention to the technical task, they had forgotten to pay attention to their patient. I was quick to remind them that this is why we run simulations and I was in no way criticising their proficiency in the technical task, but with a little more attention given to Annie other risks could be avoided alongside the danger of infection. I still remember their somewhat shocked faces as they noticed that they had briefly forgotten all about their patient, without even intending it.

Defining Risk

To begin untangling the concept of risk to consider it through an applied drama and performance lens and apply these findings back into person-centred nursing, the notion of risk needs careful definition. Following the recommendation of Battistelli and Galantino (2019), I aim to avoid using risk as a 'catch-all' and thereby offer a particular definition of risk. To be specific, I define risk as a subjective consideration of an unknown occurrence. Defining risk subjectively implies that a person's perceptions, and more pointedly their anxieties, are essential considerations when exploring risk. In this formulation, risk may be affected by and produce anxiety. Further, as Ashby and Morrell (2019) support, I assert that this subjective consideration is ever-present, 'there is always risk, it is never zero' (p. 1). Risk as it is perceived by individuals and societies is also 'constructed and thus malleable' (Orozco 2017: p. 38). It could be rightly inferred that '[i]n relation to risk, context is everything' (O'Grady 2017b: p. 5). Lash (2018) reflects on the work of prominent risk theorist Ulrich Beck, and states that over the modern era the social construction and contexts in which risk have been considered have moved 'from fated, to determinate, to indeterminate' (Lash 2018: p. 118). Although risk is often associated with danger, uncertainty or vulnerability, it is none of these things, and to avoid the conflation identified in nursing and the difference in perception based on historical and cultural contexts I intend to 'not only specify what risk is but distinguish it from what it is not' (Battistelli and Galantino 2019: p. 65).

Danger and Uncertainty

As Luhmann (1993) originally suggested, risk is not the same as danger, as outcomes from risks are internal whereas outcomes from dangers are external. For example, one of the dangers in the example of the students in their role play simulating a sterile field given above might be infection and co-infection from bacteria which are external to us. However, the risks involved are considered internally. For instance, the decision of the group to take samples is based on an internal consideration of the risk. They do not know the outcome of these actions, but see them as necessary risks. Moreover, in Beck's conception of risk as Lash (2018) clarifies, risk is defined as consequential rather than causal, which moves risk away from being the primary cause to a certain effect, whereas danger maintains a firmer link to a specific and objective outcome (p. 118). Danger as a concept is far more causal than risk. Infection is dangerous as it leads directly to harm whilst deciding to take a sample is a risk, as there are multiple potential consequences to this action. It is not hard to see how taking risky actions might lead to danger, but these risks do not necessarily lead directly to the danger we have in mind. Simply often the things which cause us harm are not the things we identify as risks.

The entangling of risk and danger creates anxiety, as every risk is foreshadowed by a lurking danger, and the potential to be harmed is more prevalent. The focus on the danger of infection had shadowed the students' consideration of the dangers to the patient's well-being and personhood. If they had considered the emotional risks with an equal weighting as the physical risks at play this may not have happened. When we distinguish the two it can be said that danger is wholly negative and risk has great potential to be positive (Battistelli and Galantino 2019: p. 65). Danger, then, is an activity or event where an external force or object is perceived to directly cause harm, where risk is the perception of consequence from an activity or event. We may take a risk, but this risk is not necessarily dangerous, especially if we mitigate the danger by creating a sterile field whilst at the same time paying closer attention to how the patient is feeling at that moment. It sounds simple, but this cognitive act of holding and attending to the person within a medical space becomes increasingly difficult the more one focuses on a biomedical approach which totalises the situation to the main danger at play. Seeing through a biomedical lens that is attempting to avoid danger, the person is reduced to their condition or designation. They are 'the cancer patient', or 'bed 22', or 'the angry one'. Their personhood is subsumed by the biomedical model's insistence that dangers lurk behind every risk we take.

The work of the students was aimed squarely at reducing the likelihood of further infection, in essence creating certainty from uncertainty. Though similar, risk represents a consideration of an unknown occurrence when one has a firm understanding of what might happen, whereas uncertainty describes a lack of surety in all aspects of the situation (Roser 2017). For example, uncertainty is an abstract notion, and it might cloud how severe a patient's infection is, just as it raises questions on the veracity of testimony given in judicial courts (Boyne 2010), or unforeseen fluctuations in exchange rate variability (Smallwood 2019) and so on. In the context of health, uncertainty not only means an abstract lack of surety, but has also come to mean a very particular moment at which risk is encountered or, to borrow a term from performance theory, uncertainty creates a liminal moment (Schechner 1985) where risk—and thereby danger—is the backdrop. Uncertainty works alongside risk, as, for instance, some risks are more or less certain than others, though tellingly uncertainty is not mutually exclusive to risk as you can take risks with certainty. For example, I may be certain that my patient understands everything I am telling them and the feeling of risk in my actions changes as a result. In this way, uncertainty can be described as a possible descriptor of a risk, but not risk itself.

More uncertain risks should produce more anxiety, but, importantly, we cannot ever remove uncertainty entirely. It is worth remembering that with relevant experience we can make the consequences of our actions feel more certain. We may know from experience that even if we feel sure that our patient understands everything and is content and comfortable, this might not necessarily be the case from the patient's perspective. We can never be fully certain about how another person is feeling. This is the importance of seeing risk as a subjective experience and interpretation of events from a person's point of view. Thanks to seeing risk as subjective, uncertainty needs to be untangled from risk in a particular way. I argue uncertainty is an adequate descriptor of risk, but that uncertainty itself should not create a moment at which risk is intensified, or seen as all-encompassing. For example, waiting for a test result might naturally produce uncertainty, but it is when this uncertainty is seen to lead to risk that anxieties significantly begin. If there are ways to reduce the sense of risk in times of uncertainty, these should be explored. In a sense, uncertainty seen as a moment of not being sure should be encouraged, but we often find this difficult as we see not knowing as inherently challenging and risky.

Vulnerability and Debility

Vulnerability has seen two main interpretations, as a universal feature of human mortality or as a feature denoting susceptibility to harm (Martin et al. 2014: p. 51–52). The former interpretation influences a move towards ethics based on the potential for all human beings to be harmed, such as the ethics of care (Gilligan 1990; Held 2006; Noddings 2013). The latter has informed the field of bioethics in determining who requires extra medical and social attention, such as the 'mentally ill and the elderly' (Ashby and Morrell 2019: p. 2). Jennings et al (2020) highlight how thinkers such as Butler (2016), 'argue for a re-evaluation of vulnerability, away from ideas of victimhood and passivity' (Jennings et al, 2020: 202). Meanwhile, drawing on Martha Fineman (2008), they state how 'far from being a state of lower status and victimhood, vulnerability is a key ontological feature of being human' (Jennings et al, 2020: 202). Professor of medical ethics Joachim Boldt describes how vulnerability is 'an all-pervasive phenomenon', which can be physical, emotional or, he crucially adds, cognitive (2019: p. 1). Boldt's addition of cognitive vulnerability means that vulnerability is not only an increased likelihood of physical or emotional harm but more precisely a 'state of physical, emotional, and cognitive stability [...] susceptible to destabilising influences' (Ibid: p. 2–3). Where risk in our definition describes our subjective perception of an unknown occurrence, vulnerability, drawing on Boldt's definition, can be defined as our potential to be destabilised—or to put it in less negative terms, the potential to be transported to a different stability. It is clear, then, that these terms are particularly resonant, as risk can make us feel vulnerable, and admitting our vulnerabilities can feel like a risk—whilst each has the potential to produce deep and interlinked feelings of anxiety. These feelings of anxiety can be a large factor in not taking a risk or avoiding feeling vulnerable.

Fidment (2012) describes how some SRP assessments cause deep anxiety in students, whilst Buxton (2011) describes how '[m]any nursing students express feelings of fear and anxiety that they will say the wrong thing' (p. 29). In our example at the start of this chapter, whether purposefully or not, students will say nothing and avoid expressing any feelings to focus on the task at hand, avoiding feeling their own—or acknowledging other people's—vulnerability. It is noteworthy that this is not based on intent as our students never intended to ignore Annie, rather it was a subconscious after-effect of the entangling of risk, danger, uncertainty, and vulnerability. I argue this stems from the students trying to manage this by focusing on their clinical task. This is an understandable outcome of a healthcare system that centres on systems that reduce risks, rather than the person at the centre of the experiences. This is the ill caused by an over-reliance on the biomedical model of health. Annie's wound must be dealt with, and creating a sterile field to do so is an excellent choice. This is an approach we should be thankful for in the biomedical model of health championing. However, person-centredness reminds us that Annie is *more than her wound.*

Vulnerability and risk both open up the perception of possibility, pathways for the future which we are unable, or perhaps less able, to predict. Where 'the cultivation of risk can be understood as a means of undermining ontological security' in ourselves and in the world around us, in moving towards vulnerability we shift from stability to instability (O'Grady 2017b: p. 9). This can be less threatening and more invitational. Vulnerability as an invitation to participate echoes Gareth White's (2013) 'Aesthetics of the Invitation', where a performer can invite audience members to become participants by, as one possible tactic, displaying vulnerability (p. 153). Taking risks and exploring vulnerability both enact a double-move, in which we challenge our perception of ourselves as fixed and stable whilst testing the actions, agency, and autonomy we ontologically perceive to have towards the environments and others we engage with. What problematizes this is when the bioethical approach described above denotes certain individuals as more or less vulnerable than others. People labelled as vulnerable are often forced into a socially and culturally constructed instability or marginalisation. This is well known within disability scholarship, where the denotation of 'disabled' is seen as a socially constructed term enforced onto people as a status marking them as 'other'. This is often referred to as the 'social model of disability' (Oliver 1983; Kuppers 2009). The notion of debility seen as a universal human condition can challenge this.

Kuppers highlights how in a biomedical model disabled people are seen as 'faulty, in need of being (and potentially able to be) cured, managed, rehabilitated' (2009: p. 225). By challenging a division between disabled and non-disabled peoples (Kuppers 2009; Goodley 2014), and advocating for a shared understanding of vulnerability as a universal factor of our existence (Fineman 2008; Butler 2016), I argue that Calvert's (2020) notion of 'debility' offers a path forward. In Calvert's model, we see 'care as fluid and mutual, constantly adjusting to the fluctuating vulnerabilities of interdependent people' (2020: p. 97). In this way, one does not ascribe the culturally unstable status of vulnerability to another, but instead we share in our mutual and relational vulnerability. We all share in the care and support that we all require to varying degrees. This opens the potential for the understanding of person-hood and agency for all bodies and all persons. In some cases, even the bodies of the mannequins we use for SRP (Tizzard-Kleister and Jennings 2020).

Untangling the Barrier Created by Risk Aversion

PCN 'represents a shift from 'one size fits all' care based on standardised data to decision-making that starts with values, expectations, preferences, relationships, hopes and fears' (McCormack et al. 2017: p. 13). The PCNF asserts that the primacy of developing competencies which aim at avoiding the danger of infection and harm—though important—should work alongside competencies aimed at building relationships, working effectively in teams, and providing holistic, effective and affective care (McCormack and McCance 2010). The PCNF argues further that 'focusing on tasks can be a defence mechanism, protecting nurses from the emotional labour of nursing work' (Ibid: p. 101). And so nurses soon become too anxious to take risks which may lead to personal growth or avoid the use of innovative methods and so on. Personal anxiety, due to conflating risk with danger, uncertainty, and vulnerability, is one barrier. Another is when workplace 'culture may prohibit the expression of practitioner vulnerability' (Wasylko and Stickley 2003: p. 446) and so stifle a practitioner's ability to perform with autonomy.

PCN recognises that the quality of care relies heavily on the care environment and the difference between culture and context in determining this. In this case, 'culture' broadly means an understanding of what actions are permitted and which ones are not by people within that culture. This means the notion of 'context' is the moment at which a person must interpret what actions are afforded to them in that given time by what they understand of the environment and culture. This therefore means that actions performed by a person within a certain context can create 'culture'. As McCormack and McCance put it, culture 'is created and recreated by the actors in the context' of a given moment, which has broader implications than that one single act (2010: p. 62). Simply, actions and behaviours propagate cultures, as much as actions and behaviours are confined, condoned, or celebrated by culture. Titchen et al. (2017) highlight a need for PCN practitioners to develop 'characteristics such as being authentically other-centred and caring, knowing self, being reflexive, patient, optimistic and open, as well as a willingness to show vulnerability' (p. 38) to be able to incite positive change and then perpetuate strong person-centred cultures. To achieve this, practitioners and students must experience vulnerability in engaging, creative, and challenging situations (Dewing and McCormack 2015: 6).

Despite the call for 'relational connectedness and the creation of psychologically safe, critical and creative communicative spaces from which emancipatory and transformative action can emerge' (Titchen et al. 2017: p. 39), there are few if any suggestions on how to teach these skills, nor ways to develop these spaces in an educational context. Moreover, a study by Dingwall et al. (2017) looked at the effect of a drama-based intervention on different healthcare practitioner's attitudes. They conclude that '[r]isk aversion' was a 'fundamental barrier to true person-centred nursing practice', where it did not seem to have been for other healthcare professions (6). The cultural perception in nursing of risk as danger and uncertainty creates anxiety in individuals and halts them from purposefully experiencing vulnerability in a way that opens them up to new experiences. Instead, the vulnerability that they are left with is bound up with feelings of danger and uncertainty with an all-pervasive riskiness affecting everything they do. To grossly oversimplify, as few 'vulnerable actions' are performed, no culture is created which embraces vulnerability as a key part of the learning experience to become person-centred.

Many seek to address this issue from the top down, instilling a culture and environment that embraces vulnerability, but this misses the need for acts of vulnerability to sustain and create these spaces. It is true, however, that acts of vulnerability on their own likewise will not achieve this aim. The lack of practical methods for developing the necessary skills and environments to challenge this 'stimulates mistrust and creates a barrier to participation and creative risk-taking' (O'Grady 2017b: 22). I argue that engagement with applied drama not only promotes the performance of vulnerable acts, but also offers a way to create a culture and environment characterised by an embrace of vulnerability, and ultimately, person-centredness. Nicholson explains how applied drama creates a space where 'people feel safe enough to take risks and to allow themselves and others to experience vulnerability' (2005: 129). 'If nursing education struggles to provide such a "safe space" for students to challenge the perception of vulnerability as a sign of "victimhood"', Jennings et al (2020 points out, 'perhaps applied drama can provide the techniques and spaces to explore the emotional risk of PCN' (p. 202). I contend that through drama, nursing students can embrace their vulnerability in safety, and thereby begin to build person-centred cultures through their collective action.

Using Drama-Based Approaches to Reframe Risk

O'Grady (2017a) examine how risk is used in contemporary performances which rely on some form of participation. For them, of key interest is performance which involves risk to create 'spaces in which participants might experience vulnerability critically' and acts as 'a deliberate aesthetic choice that foregrounds notions of openness, accountability, and trust' (2017a: p. xi). This moves away from what Dwyer et al. (2014) criticise as risk solely used for '"daring" aesthetics or "on-trend" audience engagement', and instead begins to consider how risk can be used through performance to explore 'lasting interpersonal and social consequences' (p. 1). For Spence et al. (2017) live performance creates an elevated space where sharing and engaging may be incredibly risky. However, this is a space where the act of sharing is a feature which constructs the framing of the event and cuts through the difficulties of 'open' social interaction by offering a controlled space in which to approach activities or revelations. For Hadley, this type of performance invites spectators to participate, serving to put 'the spectators' choices on display' (2017: p. 58), making the risks they take performative. Whilst it is understood that the actions of these participants do not necessarily have full real-world consequences, and the risks are less serious as a result, there is a concurrent elevation of their actions due to placing them within a participative and performative frame. It can feel like people are watching their choices, even if no one is. The participation is therefore elevated. Participants may not be acting 'as they would' in real life, but a key part of most participatory performances is how participants are asked to perform as themselves, especially when this performance occurs in 'everyday' public space. Nicholson describes how you can perform as, 'in Schechner's terms, 'not me-not not me'' (Schechner 2003: p. 270, cited in Nicholson 2005: p. 97). Participants in these types of performance are both themselves but not themselves. They are in the real world of the 'everyday', and simultaneously alongside it. They are, borrowing Baim et al.'s (2002) concept, 'one step removed' from the reality of both the world and a stable sense of self. As a result, I suggest that a performative frame is particularly suited for exploring aspects of risk in nursing contexts.

Participatory performance offers a framework through which to understand encounters with risk as 'liminal moments' (Turner 1982; Schechner 1985) we are tasked with navigating. Liminality is a term most associated with anthropology before it was made popular in performance studies by Turner (1982) and Schechner (1985) during the performative turn. In broad terms, liminality defines a moment of being in between. It is widely described as the moment at which the ephemerality of live performance is encountered and experienced. Whereas—as mentioned earlier in this chapter—encountering risk can create a liminal moment for nursing students, performance can be used purposefully to create a liminal moment within which to explore risk. This is an important distinction, as in the former risk is pervasive and a central concern as it creates the liminal moment, whereas in the former the performance frame creates a distance from risk as it becomes a subject of that liminal moment and not the creator of it. For our context of applying drama to person-centred nursing, the creation of performative encounters with risk is a powerful and necessary starting point. However, Sloan recommends we move beyond this liminal moment into co-creating an 'affective encounter that is shared, where individual embodied experience is connected with others during the inter-relation of the creation or sharing of a performance' (Sloan 2018: p. 592). Applying drama-based practices may offer methods within this frame to explore our subjective perceptions of risk and promote the co-creation of embodied and affective encounters. In these spaces, we might develop our agency through that embodiment (Nolan 2009). This is not just in the moment of performance but throughout the process of the work of drama. Following our definitions and explorations of risk in the earlier section, this frame employs risks as either physically or emotionally dangerous actions with the uncertainty of the consequences often used as a dramaturgical choice by the artist or facilitator.

For Baim (2017), discussing the risks of retelling personal narratives in applied drama work, there are different levels to engage in, each with different dangers and uncertainties at play whilst 'restaging vulnerability' (p. 100). Though this is in no way 'new news' for applied theatre practitioners, it is surprising to still find many who use drama and storytelling in applied contexts who assume that storytelling is an automatically positive activity and experience. For others, personal narratives offer an opportunity and starting point to rehearse community action. These approaches draw from Paolo Freire (2000) and Augusto Boal (1998), where 'risk is deployed as a tactic by which we learn to act and to take action in our own lives' (O'Grady 2017b: p. 15). Brodzinski defines the strategy of storytelling from the personal to the communal as 'cognitive adaptation', where 'creative activity' and 'metaphoric narrativization' act as 'a resistant tactic that gives voice to those who might usually be silenced' (2010: p. 37). Taking risks and experiencing vulnerability may be used through these frames to challenge culturally constructed ideas, particularly those which are ingrained and normalised.

I argue that engaging with performative risk-taking simulates and elevates encounters. Moreover, it moves from the personal to the communal, straddling the border between the level of context and the level of culture. At its heart, the approach aims to simulate what Brodzinski calls an 'embodied encounter', with another person who is complex and compelling as an agent in the simulated world (2010: p. 150). The frame provided by participative performance may be well suited as a frame through which to explore nursing students' abilities to perform sympathetic presence, and in a deeper way to explore and know themselves and what personhood means to them. However, to avoid this process becoming task-based, where the student 'resolves' the tensions of a specific encounter and doesn't think about it again, it is important to consider this moment beyond a singular, liminal, and momentary exchange. Instead, these moments should constitute a continuing ethic based on care. I propose that the aesthetics of care (Thompson 2015) offers a viewpoint to achieve this concerning applied drama practice. I also suggest that engaging in drama-based activity beyond a one-off event (for instance, a series of SRP developed in partnership with a drama facilitator) may lead to invigorating outcomes. As the concluding chapter of this book will argue, the best results of this will only begin to emerge if curricula are person-centred (as argued recently by a host of person-centred scholars in the creation of a person-centred curriculum framework—see Cook et al. 2022), and approaches across disciplines, such as those explored in this book offered from applied drama, help students and staff better explore person-centredness theoretically and practically.

The aesthetics of care offers a unique and new way to identify aesthetics in performance works, it also offers a way for us to use these relational affective encounters to explore risk and shared vulnerabilities. Engaging with an aesthetic of care better leads us to understand the 'lasting interpersonal and social consequences' of the art we engage in (Dwyer et al. 2014: p. 1). Hargrave makes the argument that vulnerability has aesthetic potential in how it is shared, taken up and exposed by spectators and performers in participatory performance (Hargrave, 2017). Meanwhile, Spence et al. (2017) note how their 'aesthetic performance hinged on our participants' willingness to take risks' (p. 171). Many conceptions of aesthetics in applied drama work focus on the point of performance (White 2015). This can be argued to be true of participatory and 'immersive' practices in what Machon (2013) and Shaughnessy (2015) call 'syn-aesthetics'. By adopting a relational aesthetics of care instead of an intervention being solely about an outcome it also becomes about the features of the relationships explored in and beyond that moment. By adopting this approach care, like aesthetics, is not seen as momentary or transactional, but as a process and an ethic where it is never 'finished'. The aesthetic of that care likewise is not placed in one single moment or practice but within the fabric of the care experience. Applying this to our framing of risk as performative does similar work in identifying and exposing students to risk beyond a momentary instance of danger, uncertainty, or vulnerability. Instead, students may begin to see how risk is everpresent, subjective, contextual, and constructed. Through these frameworks, care becomes an acknowledgement of ever-present risk and mutual vulnerability, and a shared debility. Meanwhile, the actions of trying to take care of myself and others relationally and affectively can be seen as a fundamental ethos underlying all of the work of nursing staff. Though these encounters with vulnerability may be uncomfortable, they powerfully tap into 'moments of critical vulnerability that put us in touch with the present and the presence of others' (O'Grady 2017b: p. 13).

Creating Spaces of Potentiality

Dwyer et al. (2014) highlight that applied theatre spaces are often assumed to be safe, they are spaces designed to cognitively separate us from the real world with a 'permeable membrane' (p. 1). However, as they also suggest, the fragility of these spaces—and the place of risk in them—is under-considered (Ibid). Applying drama can be considered a way to develop creativity (Dümenci and Keçeci 2014), and so applied drama is often considered inherently creative. However, as Gardiner (2016) argues, this assumed 'intrinsic creativity' may be halting practitioners from developing and practicing specific methods to explore further (p. 248). Organisations often seek to use drama and dramatic spaces as solutions for teaching 'uncreative' subjects. The creative potential of applied drama space is frequently assumed and co-opted (Fryer 2010; Davis 2015). Brodzinski highlights how in many theatre and health interventions the space of the 'health institution is in direct relation to the physical encounter of the theatrical event', and these interventions are often used to 'mediate difficult thoughts and feelings through creative means' (2010: p. 26, 31). This can be a positive, in that it makes the difficult parts of healthcare experiences more bearable, understandable, and beautiful. However, it is all too easy to use approaches like this to plaster over cracks in a system. In a separate project, Brodzinski exposes the way the NHS approaches creativity by trying to create 'a "failsafe toolkit"' as fundamentally uncreative (Allen and Brodzinski 2009: p. 310). The notion of a safe and/or creative space is always contestable, particularly in drama-based interventions in healthcare. Two examples from applied drama relating to the construction and utilisation of 'space' that seem particularly resonant to this study are the 'congenial' and the 'dilemmatic' space.

   White (2009) defines the congenial space as 'a climate for meaningful engagement where conversation comes naturally' (p. 105). This space is socially and psychologically safe. It is an environment that moves away from a focus on failure as entirely negative, and being incorrect as a fatal flaw. It involves promoting natural responses uninhibited by any perceived restrictions. A congenial space is both constructed purposefully as well as created live in an ephemeral moment. White (2009) describes the construction of purposefully congenial space in a project by *Roots and Wings*, where an art room is open to pupils during break times at a primary school. This 'is not just an activity room; it is a space to foster empathy and to model and analyse relationships in a child-friendly way.' This room provided 'a congenial space' to build a sense of 'connection through a supportive sense of place' as well as arts activities (Ibid: p. 192, 75).

Congenial space can also emerge between groups of people. This type of congenial space is often unprompted and unpredictable. Robson (cited in White 2009) reflects on a project in Johannesburg for early years educators, describing how the multi-national participants attempted to communicate with words and encountered difficulty. Eventually, they found a shared understanding through an improvised moment of communal singing. Although this was not the intention of the facilitators the unprompted communal singing created a congenial space in action. This was created through mutual action discovered by the group, though it was incited by a solo singer. Spence et al. (2017) describe a similar process of generous sharing by an individual that galvanises a group through performed actions. This is a process where a group supports and gives acceptance to a solo presenter through generosity. This space can be said to resonate with Carl Rogers' (1961) idea of 'unconditional positive regard' (notably, this is also a key consideration in PCN), where people are regarded positively as a first step and a priority, regardless of any other presuppositions. When one person opens up and expresses their vulnerability, a congenial space is created when those who are with them choose to care for them and share a mutual sense of vulnerability. The congenial space is fundamentally a space of acceptance and openness with few—if any—imposed limits. It is important to note that a person 'stepping up' and being vulnerable seems to be a common feature for the creation of a congenial space. In many respects, this is a brave act, and could rightly be seen as creating a brave space. This is particularly so when considering the impact of working in a dilemmatic space.

In contrast to congenial space, the dilemmatic space is unforgiving. Preston (2016) defines dilemmatic space as 'far from being affirming and supportive', but a space in which contradictory and messy cultural and political tensions act (p. 59). Through a reliance on often precarious sources of funding and working in complex areas with various organisational and personal contestations, 'dilemmatic space *is* the inevitable context of Applied Theatre work' (Ibid, emphasis in original: p. 60). Although this space is a challenging one to act and exist within, and doesn't sound suitable for use as a basis for our formulations, it does offer a unique opportunity. As Preston continues to describe, a key approach to remaining resilient within the dilemmatic space is through openness, comfort with vulnerability and the cultivation of strong relationships (2016: p. 57–85). Similar to nursing practice, it also requires active emotional labour (Hochschild 1983; Smith 1992; Tait 2021).

The concept of emotional labour has been influential in the growth of both applied drama and nursing, but the concept is not without criticism, particularly in terms of the assumption that both applied drama facilitation and practice and the work of nurses require a significant and eventually debilitating amount of emotional

labour. Low (2020) suggests that applied drama projects characterised by reciprocity do not require the assumed emotional labour from the facilitator or participant.
This echoes many in nursing who challenge the idea of emotional labour as negative, with many indicating that the emotional labour of nursing is the most rewarding, joyful, stimulating, and meaningful part of the profession. As Delgado et al.
(2017) suggest it is emotional dissonance which should be avoided, not emotional
labour. They go further to link the notion of surface acting with outcomes of burnout
and dissociation. In simple terms, the more we feel burnt out, the less deeply we act
with others, and likewise, the more we avoid acting deeply with others (think emotional labour) the more likely burnout seems to become. What this position reminds
us is it is not the emotional interactions with persons involved in what we are doing
that are necessarily producing challenging emotional dissonance. For example,
facilitating drama activities with working-class teenagers or nursing an elderly person may not involve challenging emotional labour, rather it may be the most stimulating part of the work. What is undeniably causing this difficult emotional
dissonance is the dilemmatic contexts this work has to be conducted within. It is
often the fault of other competing concerns such as a funding body's requirement
that these teenagers learn specific new behaviours, or that you have less time to
nurse your elderly patient one-to-one because staffing levels are low. A dilemmatic
space can lead one to surface acting, to not finding stimulation in the emotional
labour of one's work, to emotional dissonance, and—eventually—to burnout.

Working in a dilemmatic space also requires individuals to engage in criticality;
to constantly re-evaluate the situations they are in, their own and other's preconceptions and how they engage with people in messy contexts. This consequently creates
an environment that requires people-centred skills, reflected in how the PCNF
describes characteristics of person-centred environments, such as the 'potential for
innovation and risk-taking'. I contend that we cannot avoid the dilemmatic space
nor the taxing effect of emotional labour, regardless of how reciprocal the relationships we build, or however affective the experience is. I argue that even if the emotional labour of nursing is stimulating and joyful, at the same time, it is also often
challenging, it is tiring, and it is difficult to negotiate. It is also highly contextual,
and environment-specific. The concept of dilemmatic space shows that factors are
backgrounding the work we do, and Preston (2016) highlights the need for critical
and creative awareness of these factors to better facilitate our work. For example, do
nurses have the time to engage in emotional labour in the ways they would like
when working within a system that prioritises the efficiency of technical tasks above
all else? What applied drama and the notion of purposefully dilemmatic spaces offer
is a platform through which to explore how we might do so. Likewise, for nurses
who find emotional labour the most challenging part of their practice, dilemmatic
space used purposefully in an educational environment presents a chance to confront this and find out what it is that is making it difficult.

What we might do is redirect the dilemma and emotional labour and make them
a feature of the work. In this case, we must not shy from the inherent moral, cultural,
and emotional dilemmas, but instead position them as purposeful aspects of what
we do. In this way, we do not use drama to create an abstract situation to play

within, nor do we use drama to create high-fidelity situations to navigate. We instead engage in dramatic practice to explore complex situations that are located and 'real', above and beyond a simple mimetic representation through 'high fidelity'. What applied drama offers is a space where the contexts that background our real work can be magnified to whatever degree is necessary to identify and then address how we better negotiate them. If we consider the dilemmatic space fashioned as a democratic space, it becomes a space in which groups are purposefully challenged and provoked by a specific set of dilemmas and contexts to work through. The group must explore this collectively, dialogically, and dynamically to be successful person-centred practitioners. In a dilemmatic space, a crucial learning point to be found is that we cannot remove or control the 'vicarious response of compassion' we feel (Hepplewhite 2020: p. 66). This is exacerbated by the various systemic dilemmas permeating the environments in which we work (think understaffing, poor resources, lack of skill mix, and so on). Through engaging with dilemmas collectively we can find ways to better manage them. Drama has a history of cultivating exercises that help performers and communities do just that.

It might be possible to play out our dilemmas into an SRP or drama-based exercise to simulate a 'real' and problematic situation, with all of its fidelity, and its chaos. Returning to Spence et al. (2017), performance spaces rely on acceptance, but they also rely on a sense of dissonance. As they state, in their work 'no risk or vulnerability occurred without intimacy, and no intimacy occurred without dissonance' (p. 166). The dilemmatic space calls to attention a dissonance and engaging in that dissonance calls for a solution. This creates a space that promotes self-awareness and engaged working relationships whilst challenging assumptions, boundaries, and habits in a way which feels risky but is not necessarily dangerous. Preston (2016) highlights the need for 'a political economy of emotions' in approaching and existing in these dilemmatic spaces (p. 61). She expands by stating how doing so may give us the 'courage to be vulnerable' and how engaging in those dilemmas critically helps us to develop 'the capacity to engage, even flourish, with discomfort' (Ibid, p. 85). These skills are essential for Person-Centred Nurses to flourish in less-than-ideal care environments of all kinds, and to even be drivers of cultural change. It is also the precursor to the brave step required to be vulnerable and generous to offer something, for a group to recognise and take on and create a congenial space.

To answer PCN researchers' calls for safe spaces in which students can try out risky methods (Titchen et al. 2017), I applied a synthesis of the congenial and dilemmatic space within the intervention of this research study. By purposefully adopting an approach which draws from the acceptance and encouraged creativity of the congenial space whilst exploring and overcoming specific dilemmas through purposefully designed dilemmatic space, we may begin to create a 'space of potentiality' (Sloan 2018). Sloan (2018), drawing from Massumi's (2002) distinction between possible and potential, moves applied drama beyond tick-box exercises often set out by funding bodies as markers of a project's success, to a 'freer form of [...] the creative process' (Sloan 2018: p. 586). I theorise that in these spaces PCN students may be afforded a framework through which to challenge their personhood as formed by their habits, patterns, and boundaries. As Buxton (2011) agrees, '[b]y practicing their communication skills using drama, nurses may explore alternative approaches in a controlled and safe environment' (p. 32). In many ways, this may cultivate the bravery to be vulnerable, to take that first step in inviting others to join in creating spaces which are congenial, safe, and creative. It is, after all, people who create the environments for the flourishing of others, it is people who must create the spaces we seek to be characterised by person-centredness, compassion, and care.

This drama-based pedagogical methodology therefore offers PCN students the opportunity to explore the potential of their personhood in an environment which is congenial in accepting how you approach uncomfortable dilemmas. This describes the key relationships across the different levels of the PCNF. For example, environments that excel at the characteristics described in the PCNF are more likely to facilitate nurses to explore how they might build the pre-requisites and perform the processes required of a person-centred nurse. It also offers a space which re-configures aesthetics to be found in the shape and sensation of relationships, and so care explored within this framework becomes both an ethical and aesthetic engagement with others. This crucially moves person-centredness away from a recognition of self as static (i.e., self as a fixed identity made up of 'competencies' and 'attributes' which are immutable) to one where self is fluid and relational (i.e., one where identity is defined by actions, interactions, and intra-actions). Extending the congenial and dilemmatic space beyond a framed encounter with risk in a simulated moment, and into an aesthetics of care, potentially creates an embodied experience to promote person-centred practice for PCN students. This may encourage PCN students 'to look anew at what they think they know and so allow a space for potentiality to emerge' (Sloan 2018: p. 591) in the care environments they act within, the relationships they build and in their sense of personhood. This is the perfect starting point from which to develop an understanding and practice of sympathetic presence as relational through performativity.

Performing Person-Centred Care

Though the notion of authenticity has seen much attention in PCN studies, it seems little consideration is given to authenticity as a relational and performative concept as described in the section above. For example, McCormack and McCance (2010) highlight the importance of authenticity when considering the personhood of others to find the authentic self of that person. This implies that a performed—inauthentic—self might be less desirable or relevant to their needs. Meanwhile, other PCN researchers have touched on the importance of ensuring authenticity in how one approaches and interacts with others, 'such as being authentically other-centred and caring' (Titchen et al. 2017: p. 38)—this time implying that one might struggle to care or be other-centred without authenticity. Lastly, Hummelvoll et al. (2015) highlight how Freire's notion of authenticity as aiding people to become 'beings for themselves' influenced PCN (p. 5). Moreover, they describe how this version of authentic 'human-ness' 'emerges through invention and reinvention, and the continuing, hopeful inquiry that human beings pursue in the world, with the world, and with each other' (Ibid). This notion speaks towards a relationality and fluid sense of an authentic self. What this conception misses, by focusing on the concept of persons discovering an authentic autonomy as 'beings for themselves', is the necessity of others to support this singular 'being', and the interrelated necessity of multiple—performed—selves in creating a 'singular' person. This is both for internal selves and external selves. Simply, one's ever-changing sense of self and others one encounters. The term 'beings for themselves' misses the importance of 'other selves' in creating, sustaining, evolving, and challenging a singular 'being'.

There is an appreciation in PCN for understanding '[c]aring as an affect' which, according to McCormack and McCance (2010), 'emphasises the nature of the emotional involvement in caring' (p. 25). However, in this case, affect is linked closely with emotion. Drama-based scholars such as Nicholson (2017) and Tait (2021) differentiate emotion and affect. For Nicholson, 'emotion can be identified, registered, and captured, whereas affects are experienced less consciously on a visceral, sensed and embodied level, moving biopolitically between human and nonhuman materialities' (2017: p. 108). I argue that both of the areas identified above may be due to PCN's humanist and individualist underpinnings. Often, authenticity—as PCN describes it—is based on a Rogerian concept of personhood in an individualist sense. Hummelvoll et al. (2015) suggest that person-centredness as Carl Rogers theorised 'can be seen as radical for its attempts to give the person the central position and challenge bureaucracy and hierarchies in promoting the ideal of humans relating as equals' (p. 2). This move towards an equality of treatment for humans denotes a sense of universality of personhood. However, the idiosyncratic nature of human perception and socialisation causes friction when considering what is (socially) deemed personhood and what is not. As Nolan argues, what is 'socially sanctioned' affects the 'material body', but when we experience new bodily sensations and affects we might challenge this (2009: p. 28). Through this, we can see how personhood can be affected, and that PCN does not necessarily encourage an entirely individualist approach, though it would often seem so from some of the language used in PCN theory. Even by its terminology that (literally) centres people, person-centeredness might be considered to be a process of individuation or rather personalisation. What is clear from the discussion, utilisation, and application of the theory into practice is that this is not necessarily always the case.

Many PCN researchers move away from certain individualistic essentialisms. For instance, Dewing et al. (2017) draw on Buber's 'I-thou'/ 'I-It' concept—where, crudely, an 'I-Thou' relationship describes a relationship between two entities who are closer to being peers more often associated with human-to-human relationships, and an 'I-It' relationship is one between, say, a person and a thing, where the relationship is less balanced in terms of power between these entities. Dewing et al explain how 'each Thou must sometimes turn into an It in relation' (2017: p. 26). Jacobs et al. (2017) recognise the criticism of Rogerian personhood as 'individualistic and decontextualised', instead they draw attention to the work of Paolo Freire as having 'laid the ground for including relational empowerment and social justice as a core element in person-centred practice' (p. 51).

It is important to examine philosophical perspectives on how reality is understood in this context. For example, if reality, as the PCN denotes personhood, is dependent on reasoning then persons with dementia would be considered less active in the world, and *less of* a person than others. They would be less able to participate in what denotes personhood as their reason diminishes or shifts, however, this runs counter to PCN beliefs and values. Skovdahl & Dewing remind us that '[o]ver and above theorising, person-centredness is a human ethical presence' (2017: p. 88). I argue, along with Mermikides (2020), that posthumanism offers a potent area for exploration regarding nursing—and PCN in particular. This is seen starkly when considering the role of non-humans in nursing care. In this example, the role of mannequins in SRPs can be seen in ways anew through performance, applied puppetry, and new materialisms (Tizzard-Kleister and Jennings 2020; Smith 2015; Mermikides 2020). As summarised in Tizzard-Kleister and Jennings (2020), applying these ideas to inanimate mannequins forces us to metaphorically translate the experience of an object to what we can understand, lighting a path for them to play all of the complexity and interdependencies of personhood through their language in an interactive SRP. This brings up questions of which bodies are more or less authentic than others, and what makes them so. Is it their capacity? Their approximate 'human-ness'? Their responsivity? These questions are expansive, and touch at the very core of the question; what is it that makes us human, and what is it that denotes us as people? It is a small leap from a speculative theorisation that through the performed personhood of objects, all personhood is intrinsically performed. This challenges the idea that personhood is non-universal.

Exploring these areas helps to flesh out and develop how a person-centred nurse might identify their own—and other's—'narrative identity'. In this way, a narrative identity will be 'recognised by the various roles played out' (McCormack and McCance 2010: p. 133). It is important to remember that the powerful contribution of a performance-based viewpoint alongside PCN is, as Conroy suggests, in how in performance '[s]elves are relational and narrative forms. The process of telling the story is a transformational event. It is not a process for relating a static set of truths to the audience' (2017: p. 100). Weaving these notions into the PCN concept of narrative identity, for instance, reveals how recognising and identifying this narrative identity is not identifying the entirety of one's identity, but the presentation of this identity in that given moment. We enter into the 'stories' of those we meet at that moment, we can't know their whole story in that first meeting. Moreover, we are always an outside interpreter of the 'narrative identities', or stories, of others. Tizzard-Kleister and Jennings (2020) remind us that interactions based on transactions are assumptive and that we can learn processes of translation through non-humans which can aid us in developing skills at translating the personhood of humans. It may be, then, that looking at the non-human may help us to interact and relate to the human in a more person-centred way. This poses another challenge to the assumed individuating nature of PCN's humanism and notion of the authentic as an essentialism. As Spence et al. (2017) put it, when performance-based approaches which performatively frame notions of risk and participation are then applied to other disciplines 'non-professionals may be guided towards a more 'cultural', 'high intensity', 'formal', 'conscious', 'high risk', and/or 'high reward' […] experience' of 'powerfully felt but somewhat nebulous affective states' (p. 158). In these cases, PCN might gain useful perspectives and positions from which to build robust educational practices, drawn from the long histories of drama-based areas which move beyond static ideas of personhood.

Person-Centred Care as Facilitation

Lieshout and Cardiff (2015) draw parallels between PCN and facilitation and attempt to define what person-centred facilitation might be. They summate that it 'is not just about helping others to change their current situation. It is also about being attentive to the personhood of others and self, embedded within complex and dynamic contexts' (Lieshout and Cardiff 2015: p. 8). This is extraordinarily resonant with applied drama approaches to facilitation (Preston 2016; Hepplewhite 2020). As applied drama facilitation expert, Sheila Preston (2016) describes, '[a] resilient and mindful approach aligned with a critical facilitation practice can provide us with the capacity to notice and engage with what is happening in the room' (Preston 2016: p. 85). Meanwhile, Hepplewhite (2020) advocates for the term 'applied theatre artist' over facilitator, though recognises that regardless of title, good practice relies on 'attunement' and 'responsivity' with others. I argue that these resonant approaches should be considered alongside one another, where the particular contexts of PCN influence the critical approach for applied drama practices whilst the experienced interactive pedagogy of applied drama might influence how PCN is taught.

In a rare example of drama used to enhance person-centred approaches, Kontos et al. (2010) highlight how drama can help to practically achieve PCN objectives by, for instance, emphasising 'the importance of using knowledge of the particularities of the resident to identify patterns of behaviour to reveal unmet needs' (p. 160). Jennings et al (2020) suggest this is difficult for a student nurse to do when working in a 'mechanistic' paradigm (de Zulueta 2013: p. 123), and when facing a staffing crisis (Louch et al. 2016). Many projects rely on enhancing healthcare students and staff's capacity for empathy to avoid this (Eisenberg et al. 2015; Yakhforoshha et al. 2017). PCN and the PCNF in particular are more critical of empathy as it relates to nursing. McCormack and McCance (2010) advocate for sympathetic presence over empathy. They describe how one cannot 'fully comprehend another individual's particular experience' (p. 102), and as empathy asks us to do just that it is 'neither desirable nor possible' (Jennings et al, 2020: 192). What drama can help to reveal are the subtexts and features behind what Kontos et al. (2010) called 'patterns of behaviour' (p. 160) to help understand others through their actions—or rather their performances of their 'self'. This moves away from understanding others through empathy, instead we understand them through their interpersonal actions.

Authenticity, the Dramaturgy of Everyday Life, Performativity and PCN

Goffman (1990) defines the self in everyday life as reliant on presentation, on the intention behind an action or bodily presence and the subsequent interpretation of this action. This is 'a kind of information game', where one might consider the information dramaturgically in 'a potentially infinite cycle of concealment, discovery, false revelation, and rediscovery' (Goffman 1990: p. 20). Goffman's sociological theory has been applied to a variety of contexts, not least back to drama. Goffman's notion was a key part of what is called 'the performative turn', the most prominent proponent of which is Richard Schechner (1985, 2003). Broadly, this opened out the focus of drama studies to consider a wider and more eclectic range of stimuli and approaches to performing in and beyond the theatre. As Brodzinski (2014) states, '[c]ontemporary dramatic practice has problematized the relationship between art and everyday life' (p. 165). In many cases, performance studies became a critique of theatre and drama as an apparatus. For instance, the role of the performer after the performative turn is opened out, where the performer's performance 'on-stage' is considered more closely to their real life. No longer aiming exclusively to represent a character as realistically as possible on stage they are 'both performer who lives in the moment and spectator who observes and critiques the presentation' (Brodzinski 2010: p. 144). This self-consciousness purposefully draws attention to the inauthenticity of traditional, mimetic, drama-based approaches as just that—a representation of reality and not reality itself. Instead, performance studies seek to access something more 'genuine', something ephemeral, and emergent. At its heart, the performative turn can be said to aim to capture an immediate sense of action through a critique of representative action, by colliding performative elements from both everyday life and the stage. Returning to the exploration in Chap. 3, performance studies tend to move away from 'acting', and systems for actor training such as Stanislavski's MoPA. It may be the performative turn which has left Stanislavski's idea untapped by applied drama theorists and practitioners. In applied drama, there is a focus on performativity over acting. Hughes et al. (2011) define 'performative' as 'statements and actions that bring about social and material effects' (p. 201). Though it can be argued that this is a more authentic mode of performance as Nicholson (2017) reminds us, '[c]laims about authenticity are always problematic in debates about theatre' (p. 116). This is particularly so, as many contemporary examples consciously create uncertainty to challenge the notion of authenticity in the first place. This is often a productive tension rather than a roadblock.

For Boal, this was the perfect prism through which to present a spectator with ways to engage with their reality differently through the use of performance. Boal (1992) encouraged engaging in an aesthetic version of reality whilst remembering and applying the experience to one's own lived experience. He called this 'metaxis'. Metaxis is the collision of 'the image of reality and the reality of the image' (Boal 1992: p. 13). In this collision, a participant cannot be passive and must 'encounter with the space between' these worlds (Baim 2017: p. 99). Stanislavski's approaches are less considered as synergetic methods to apply a performative frame, yet

Stanislavski 'was arguably the first acting practitioner to look at what human beings do naturally in their everyday lives and turn it into something systematic for the stage' (Merlin 2014: p. 1). In essence, his ideas were intended for a particular aesthetic frame of representational mimetic acting and so have perhaps been ignored by performance studies. Through the dramaturgy of everyday life, metaxis and Stanislavski's 'magic if' can be understood to provide a position and practice to access a performative co-existence between the real and the aesthetic. Echoing Thompson's 'care aesthetics' (2015, 2023), we might also use this approach to see the aesthetics in care and care as an aesthetic. It is worth noting Stanislavski's influence on Boal, and that some make the argument that many of Boal's ideas and approaches are natural extensions of Stanislavski's ideas and approaches (Bezerra 2015). Stanislavski highlights the necessity of imagination in doing this, as '[f]rom the moment of the appearance of [the Magic] If the actor passes from the plane of actual reality into the plane of another life, created and imagined by him' (Stanislavski 1990: p. 94). What this offers for nursing education is a crucible in which to encounter and experiment, a space of potentiality (Sloan 2018) to develop and engage in sympathetic presence.

A New Perspective on Sympathetic Presence and Engagement

I argue that reconsidering the PCNF processes of 'engagement' and 'sympathetic presence' through Preston's (2016) suggestions for facilitative practice may offer an insight into how a method may be developed to encourage a changed perspective on risk. This might also offer practical methods to teach and present the skills and sustain the person-centred environments called for by PCN researchers. Preston suggests that though the facilitator feels they should adopt 'a performed neutrality', they cannot 'stand outside of the work' and so instead of being distant, passive or overly objective, must be present and 'attempt to understand the moments that emerge for us—in their complexity, messiness and difficulty—without letting our ego result in an unwitting reframing of the work around our sensitivities and sensibilities' (2016: p. 29).

Sympathetic presence is a process from the PCNF in which a practitioner acknowledges the other's personhood when compared with the self in a caring interaction. Sympathetic presence is 'more than simply being physically present' (McCance et al, 2021), it is a recognition of and emotional availability to another person (McCormack 2001a, b; McCance 2003). It also reflects a conscious move away from the problematic idea of empathy (McCormack and McCance 2010, 2016). 'Empathy requires effort' and burnout is more likely when over-empathising. Healthcare staff need support to maintain self-awareness of the 'delicate psychological balance between detachment and connection' whilst empathising with others, particularly in intense situations (Jeffrey 2017: p. 268). Sympathetic presence, conversely, allows the nurse to respect the individuality of the other without dipping into 'emotional reserves'. As mentioned in previous chapters, sympathetic presence relates to compassion more than empathy, and encouraging a presence alongside the concept of sympathy promotes what could be called compassionate action. Moreover, sympathetic presence reframes the emotional labour undertaken to understand and relate to another person, particularly when working in difficult circumstances. It is a process that guards against surface acting and avoids emotional dissonance. By considering the uniqueness of the other's emotions, we thereby remain available to relate on an emotional and rational level with others in a given—often dilemmatic—circumstance.

Sympathetic presence, however, is not so clearly described by PCN researchers. It is described as both a having (McCormack and McCance 2010: 100), a showing (Lieshout and Cardiff 2015), and a being (McCormack and McCance 2016). This confusion illustrates a lack of definitional specificity and leads to confusion which makes it difficult to find a coherent approach in which to teach it as a theoretical process, let alone demonstrate it as a practice. I argue that sympathetic presence is best described not as something we show, have or be, but as something we perform and feel. As a result, it is a process which can be taught experientially and trained for any situation, between any persons. It is further argued that Stanislavski's MoPA and other drama-based approaches might contribute to this. Considered in this way, sympathetic presence is an affirmation of each person's autonomy and interdependency through face-to-face performances of care. It is also a realisation of the near limitless creativity possible in the agency of the self; both for the nurse and, often through careful inter-relational facilitation, for the patient. This is not 'a performed neutrality' (Preston 2016: p. 29). It is a performed presence characterised by sympathy and care. This is not a performance as a lie, as a pretence of sympathy in an aloof and pretended presence. It is rather a performance of presence as a skilled and purposeful act that continually recognises and distinguishes the feelings of others and your own in greater detail.

Engagement, another named process from the PCNF, has only recently been explored in nursing, and generally aims to 'engender trust and so enable people to work together more effectively' (Dewing and McCormack 2015: p. 2). In a power relation dynamic, trust asks us whether we will serve others or ourselves. 'This also means vulnerability is a prerequisite to trust' (Dewing et al. 2017: p. 26) Alice O'Grady (2017b) describes how trust is key for participatory performance also, as 'participants enter the unfamiliar using trust' (p. 1). Moreover, commitment to being engaged can be a re-energising and vulnerable experience, and 'can be the key to unlocking productivity and potential' (Dewing and McCormack 2015: p. 6). When care focuses on 'the interaction with that person at that time' it is described as engaged (McCormack and McCance 2010: p. 97). Though engagement also refers to more than interactions between people, it also describes our relationship with the world as we open ourselves up to it. As Titchen et al. (2017) put it, when we risk engaging in the world around us 'we fall into the beauty, mystery and energy of the natural world and see the messages there for us' (p. 40). I argue for a reimagining of the term engagement as it is presented in the PCNF and imbue it with the idea of attention and generosity, particularly when considering the role of the performer and/or practitioner. It is not the 'amount' or 'depth' of attention in engaging with others that is most meaningful, but the generosity with which this is offered that creates the most potential for affect. It is the brave person who steps up, attending to and offering something to the others and to the space around them, inviting us into a—we hope—congenial space. This is often a person who steps up to do something different, or risky, in order to challenge the status quo, or advocate for others in a challenging situation. This is reminiscent of '[t]he gift of applied drama', as Helen Nicholson (2005) articulates, which 'offers an opportunity for an ethical praxis that disrupts horizons, in which new insights are generated and where the familiar might be seen, embodied and represented from alternative perspectives and different points of view' (p. 167). Engagement is then the generosity of one person's offer and attention towards another, or to their environments. It is the openness with which we encounter risk and experience ours and others' vulnerability and can be said to help produce the sympathetic presence performed and embodied by the practitioner, and a congenial space within a dilemmatic space. Engagement and sympathetic presence, then, are close bedfellows in our conceptual frame, with the notion of generosity and attention being key shared features.

Summarising the Shared Conceptual Frame

This chapter concludes Part 1 of this book and represents the creation and exploration of a shared conceptual framing between applied drama and person-centred nursing. This chapter has brought the strands woven in the previous chapters together, and suggested some conceptual threads. In this chapter, the impact of generosity and attention on the concepts of sympathetic presence and engagement has been recognised. Facilitative practice in spaces of potentiality where the congenial and dilemmatic converge have been suggested as potent spaces for creating person-centred practitioners. The notion of risk as subjective, and framed through performance practice and theory, has helped to suggest a way applied drama might encourage the necessary risk taking for person-centred practice to be taught and to flourish. The conceptual framework as a whole is difficult to summarise, but a few key features shine through. Perhaps the main feature of applying drama to person-centred nursing on this conceptual level through my work is seeing sympathetic presence anew. In this framing, sympathetic presence is *performative*. It is relational, contextual, and a process which girds person-centred practice in the interactive and inter-relational encounters between persons. What is also hopefully clear is how applied drama can offer practical approaches to teaching and practicing the performance of sympathetic presence and other person-centred processes, whilst going some way to encouraging the creation of person-centred environments and spaces for learning.

The next part of this book shifts focus. Part 2 will explore and discuss the four key themes from my doctoral study in four separate chapters. Each chapter will focus on one theme and will draw from the conceptual frame created here (just as the creation of the drama course created as part of the primary research I conducted did) as well as the results from the study. These results are drawn from qualitative data collected from the study. These data include field notes taken by me in the role of participant–observer, the participant's reflections collected through an approach

I call 'creative personal reflection', and lastly, through a focus group interview with the group. These data are presented verbatim, and fuel the discussion of how the conceptual frame was applied in this practice, finding new resonances, different paths, and more vibrant depth to the framework. By the end of this, I hope to have presented a compelling approach to interdisciplinary practice that argues for a dynamic and dyadic relationship between concept and practice in nursing and drama.

References

Allen V, Brodzinski E (2009) Deconstructing the toolkit: creativity and risk in the NHS workforce. Health Care Anal 17:309–317

Ashby M, Morrell B (2019) To your good health! Going to the pub with friends, nursing dying patients, and 'ER' receptionists: the ubiquitous rise of risk management and maybe a 'prudential' bioethics? Bioeth Inq 16:1–5

Baim C (2017) The drama spiral: a decision making model for safe, ethical, and flexible practice when incorporating personal stories in applied theatre and performance. In: O'Grady A (ed) Risk, participation, and performance practice: critical vulnerabilities in a precarious world. Palgrave Macmillan, London, pp 79–109

Baim C, Brookes S, Mountford A (2002) The geese theatre handbook: Drama with offenders and people at risk. Waterside Press, Winchester

Battistelli F, Galantino MG (2019) Dangers, risks and threats: an alternative conceptualization to the catch-all concept of risk. Curr Sociol 67(1):64–78

Bezerra AP (2015) Truth on stage, truth in life: Boal and Stanislavski. Rev Bras Estud Presença 5:2. Available from; https://www.scielo.br/scielo.php?pid=S2237-26602015000200413&script=sci_arttext&tlng=en. Accessed 14 Sept 2020

Boal A (1992) Games for actors and non-actors. Routledge, London

Boal A (1998) Theatre of the oppressed. Pluto Press, London

Boldt J (2019) The concept of vulnerability in medical ethics and philosophy. Philos Ethics Humanit Med 14(6):1–8

Boyne SM (2010) Uncertainty and the search for truth at trial: defining prosecutorial "objectivity" in German sexual assault cases. Wash Lee Law Rev 67(4):1287–1359

Brodzinski E (2010) Theatre in health and care. Basingstoke, Palgrave

Brodzinski E (2014) Performance anxiety the relationship between social and aesthetic drama in medicine and health. In: Bates V, Bleakley A, Goodman S (eds) Medicine, health and the arts: approaches to the medical humanities. Routledge, Abingdon, pp 165–185

Butler J (2016) Frames of war: when is life grievable? Verso, London

Buxton B (2011) Interaction, unscripted: an effective use of drama to simulate the nurse-client relationship. J Psychol Nurs 49(5):28–32

Calvert D (2020) Convivial theatre: care and debility in collaborations between non-disabled and learning disabled theatre makers. In: Stuart Fisher A, Thompson J (eds) Performing care: new perspectives on socially engaged performance. Manchester University Press, Manchester, pp 85–102

Conroy C (2017) Participation, recognition and political space. In: Harpin A, Nicholson H (eds) Performance and participation: practices, audiences, politics. Red Globe, London, pp 82–102

Cook NF, Brown D, O'Donnell D, McCance T, Dickson C, Tønnesen S, Dunleavy S, Lorber M, Falkenberg H, Byrne G, McCormack B (2022) The person-centred curriculum framework: a universal curriculum framework for person-centred healthcare practitioner education. Int Pract Dev J 12(4):1–11

Davis S (2015) Drama, education and curriculum: alive, kicking and counting. Res Drama Educ : Journal of Applied Theatre and Performance 20(3):327–330

de Zulueta P (2013) Compassion in 21st century medicine: is it sustainable? Clin Ethics 8(4):119–128

Delgado C, Upton D, Ranse K, Furness T, Foster K (2017) Nurses' resilience and the emotional labour of nursing work: an integrative review of empirical literature. Int J Nurs Stud 70:71–88

Dewing J, McCormack B (2015) Engagement: a critique of the concept and its application to person-centred care. Int Pract Dev J. [Online] Available from: https://www.fons.org/Resources/Documents/Journal/Vol5Suppl/IPDJ_05(suppl)_06.pdf. Accessed 13 Mar 2018

Dewing J, Eide T, McCormack B (2017) Philosophical perspectives on person-centredness for healthcare research. In: McCormack B, Dulmen S, Eide H, Skovdahl K, Eide T (eds) Person-centred nursing research. Wiley Blackwell, Chichester, pp 19–30

Dingwall L, Fenton J, Kelly TB, Lee J (2017) Sliding doors: did drama-based inter-professional education improve the tensions round person-centred nursing and social care delivery for people with dementia: a mixed method exploratory study. Nurse Educ Today 51:1–7

Dümenci SB, Keçeci A (2014) Creative drama: can it be used in nursing education. Int J Hum Sci 11(2):1320–1326

Dwyer P, Hunter MA, Pearson JS (2014) High stakes: performance and risk [editorial]. About Perf 12(1):1–5

Eisenberg A, Rosenthal S, Schlussel Y (2015) Medicine as a performing art: what we can learn about empathetic communication from theatre arts. Acad Med 90(3):272–276

Fidment S (2012) The objective structured clinical exam (OSCE): a qualitative study exploring the health care student's experience. Stud Engagement Exp J 1(1):1–18

Fineman M (2008) The vulnerable subject: anchoring equality in the human condition. Yale J Law Femin 20(1):1–25

Freire P (2000) Pedagogy of the oppressed. Continuum, New York

Fryer N (2010) From reproduction to creativity and the aesthetic towards an ontological approach to the assessment of devised performance. Res Drama Educ : The Journal of Applied Theatre and Performance 15(4):547–562

Gardiner P (2016) Playwriting pedagogy and the myth of intrinsic creativity. Res Drama Educ. The Journal of Applied Theatre and Performance 21(2):247–262

Gilligan C (1990) In a different voice: psychological theory and women's development. Harvard University Press, Cambridge MA

Goffman E (1990) The presentation of self in everyday life. Penguin, London

Goodley D (2014) Disability studies. Routledge, Oxford

Hadley B (2017) Putting prejudices on the spot and in the spotlight: the risks of politically motivated public space performance practices. In: O'Grady A (ed) Risk, participation, and performance practice: critical vulnerabilities in a precarious world. Palgrave Macmillan, London, pp 57–78

Hargrave M (2017) Dance with a stranger: Torque Show's Intimacy (2014) and the experience of Vulnerability in Performance and Spectatorship, in Risk, participation, and performance practice: Critical vulnerabilities in a precarious world, ed. A. O'Grady, Palgrave Macmillan: London, pp. 113–130.

Held V (2006) The ethics of care: personal, political, and global. Oxford University Press, Oxford

Hepplewhite K (2020) The applied theatre artist: responsivity and expertise in practice. Palgrave Macmillan, London

Hochschild AR (1983) The managed heart. University of California Press, Berkeley

Hughes J, Kidd J, McNamara C (2011) The usefulness of mess: artistry, improvisation and decomposition in the practice of research in applied theatre. In: Kershaw B, Nicholson H (eds) Research methods in theatre and performance, pp 186–209

Hummelvoll J, Karlsson B, Borg M (2015) Recovery and person-centredness in mental health services: roots of the concepts and implications for practice. Int Pract Dev J 5. Available from: https://www.fons.org/Resources/Documents/Journal/Vol5Suppl/IPDJ_05(suppl)_07.pdf. Accessed 15 Mar 2018

Jacobs G, Lieshout F, Borg M, Ness O (2017) Being a person-centred researcher: principles and methods for doing research in a person-centred way. In: McCormack B, Dulmen S, Eide H, Skovdahl K, Eide T (eds) Person-centred healthcare research. Wiley Blackwell, Chichester, pp 51–60

Jeffrey D (2017) Communicating with a human voice: developing a relational model of empathy. J R Coll Physicians Edinb 47(3):266–270

Jennings M, Deeny P, Tizzard-Kleister K (2020) Acts of Care: applied drama, 'sympathetic presence' and person- centred nursing in Stuart Fisher A, Thompson J (eds). Performing Care: New Perspectives on Socially Engaged Performance, Manchester University Press: Manchester, pp. 187–203.

Kontos PC, Mitchell G, Mistry B, Ballon B (2010) Using drama to improve person-centred dementia care. Int J Older People Nursing 5(2):159–168

Kuppers P (2009) Toward a Rhizomatic model of disability: poetry, performance, and touch. J Lit Cult Disabil Stud 1(3):221–240

Lash S (2018) Introduction: Ulrich Beck: risk as indeterminate modernity. Theory Cult Soc 35(7):117–129

Lieshout F, Cardiff S (2015) Reflections on being and becoming a person-centred facilitator. Int Pract Dev J 5. Available from: https://www.fons.org/library/journal/volume5-person-centredness-suppl/article4. Accessed 9 Mar 2018

Louch G, O'Hara J, Gardner P, O'Connor DB (2016) The daily relationships between staffing, safety perceptions and personality in hospital nursing: a longitudinal on-line diary study. Int J Nurs Stud 59:27–37

Low K (2020) Applied theatre and sexual health communication: apertures of possibility. Palgrave Macmillan, London

Luhmann N (1993) Risk: a sociological theory. de Gruyter, New York

Machon J (2013) Immersive theatres: intimacy and immediacy in contemporary performance. Palgrave Macmillan, Basingstoke

Martin AK, Tavaglione N, Hurst S (2014) Resolving the conflict: clarifying vulnerability in health care ethics. Kennedy Inst Ethics J 24(1):51–72

Massumi B (2002) Parables for the virtual: movement, affect, sensation. Duke University Press, Durham

McCance T (2003) Caring in nursing practice: the development of a conceptual framework. Res Theory Nurs Pract 17(2):101–116

McCance T, McCormack B, Tizzard-Kleister K, Wallace L (2021) Being sympathetically presence, in Fundamentals of Person-Centred Healthcare Practice, eds McCormack B, McCance T, Bulley C, McMillan A, Martin S, Brown D. Wiley-Blackwell: Chichester.

McCormack B (2001a) Autonomy and the relationship between nurses and older people. Ageing Soc 21(4):417–446

McCormack B (2001b) Negotiating partnerships with older people: a person centred approach. Ashgate Aldershot, Burlington, VT

McCormack B, McCance T (2010) Person-centred nursing: theory and practice. Wiley-Blackwell, Chichester

McCormack B, McCance T (eds) (2016) Person-centred practice in nursing and health care, 2nd edn. Wiley-Blackwell, Chichester

McCormack B, McCance T, Dulmen S, Eide H, Skovdahl K (eds) (2017) Person-centred healthcare research. Wiley-Blackwell, Chichester

Merlin B (2014) The complete Stanislavski toolkit. Nick Hern, New York

Mermikides A (2020) Performance, medicine and the human. Methuen Drama, London

Nicholson H (2005) Applied drama: the gift of theatre. Palgrave, Basingstoke

Nicholson H (2017) Affective Labours of cultural participation. In: Harpin A, Nicholson H (eds) Performance and participation: practices, audiences, politics. Palgrave Macmillan, London, pp 105–127

Noddings N (2013) Freire, Buber, and care ethics on dialogue in teaching. In: Lake R, Kress T, Giroux H, Aronowitz S, Freire P, McLaren P (eds) Paulo Freire's intellectual roots: towards historicity in praxis. Bloomsbury, London, pp 89–100

Nolan C (2009) Agency and embodiment: performing gestures/producing cultures. Harvard University Press, Harvard

O'Grady A (ed) (2017a) Risk, participation, and performance practice: critical vulnerabilities in a precarious world. Palgrave Macmillan, London

O'Grady A (2017b) Introduction: risky aesthetics, critical vulnerabilities, and edgeplay: tactical performances of the unknown. In: O'Grady A (ed) Risk, participation and performance practice: critical vulnerabilities in a precarious world. Palgrave Macmillan, London, pp 1–29

Oliver M (1983) Social work with disabled people. Macmillan, Basingstoke

Orozco L (2017) Theatre in the age of uncertainty: memory, technology, and risk in Simon McBurney's *The encounter* and Robert Lepage's *88*. In: O'Grady A (ed) Risk, participation and performance practice: critical vulnerabilities in a precarious world. Palgrave Macmillan, London, pp 33–55

Preston S (2016) Applied theatre: facilitation: pedagogies, practices, resistance. Bloomsbury Methuen, London

Rogers C (1961) On becoming a person, a therapist's view of psychotherapy. Houghton-Mifflin, Boston

Roser D (2017) The irrelevance of the risk-uncertainty distinction. Sci Eng Ethics 23:1387–1407

Schechner R (1985) Between theatre and anthropology. University of Pennsylvania Press, Pennsylvania

Schechner R (2003) Performers and spectators transported and transformed. In: Auslander P (ed) Performance: critical concepts in literary and cultural studies. Routledge, London, pp 263–290

Shaughnessy N (2015) Applying performance: live art, socially engaged theatre and affective practice. Palgrave Macmillan, London

Skovdahl K, Dewing J (2017) Co-creating flourishing research practices through person-centred research: a focus on persons living with dementia. In: McCormack B, Dulmen S, Eide H, Skovdahl K (eds) Person-centred healthcare research. Wiley-Blackwell, Chichester, pp 85–94

Sloan C (2018) Understanding spaces of potentiality in applied theatre. Res Drama Educ : The Journal of Applied Theatre and Performance 23(4):582–597

Smallwood A (2019) Analyzing exchange rate uncertainty and bilateral export growth in China: a multivariate GARCH-based approach. Econ Model 82:332–344

Smith P (1992) The emotional labour of nursing: its impact on interpersonal relations, management and educational environments. Palgrave, Basingstoke

Smith M (2015) The practice of applied puppetry: antecedents and tropes. Res Drama Educ. The Journal of Applied Theatre and Performance 20(4):531–536

Spence J, Andrews S, Frohlick D (2017) *Collect yourself*: risk, intimacy, and dissonance in intermedial performance. In: O'Grady A (ed) Risk, participation, and performance practice: critical vulnerabilities in a precarious world. Palgrave Macmillan, London, pp 153–175

Stanislavski C (1990) An actor's handbook. Methuen, London

Tait P (2021) Theory for theatre studies: emotion. Methuen drama, London

Thompson J (2015) Towards an aesthetics of care. Res Drama Educ : The Journal of Applied Theatre and Performance 20(4):430–441

Thompson J (2023) Care aesthetics: for artful care and careful art. Routledge, London

Titchen A, Cardiff S, Biong S (2017) The knowing and being of person-Centred research practice across worldviews: an epistemological and ontological framework. In: McCormack B, Dulmen S, Eide H, Skovdahl K (eds) Person-centred healthcare research. Wiley-Blackwell, Chichester, pp 31–51

Tizzard-Kleister K, Jennings M (2020) "Breath, belief, focus, touch": applied puppetry in simulated role play for person-centred nursing education. Appl Theatre Res 8(1):73–87

Turner V (1982) From ritual to theatre: the human seriousness of play. PAJ Publications, New York

Wasylko Y, Stickley T (2003) Theatre and pedagogy: using drama in mental health nurse education. Nurse Educ Today 23:443–448

White M (2009) Arts development in community health: a social tonic. Radcliffe, Oxford

White G (2013) Audience participation in theatre: aesthetics of the invitation. Palgrave Macmillan, London

White G (2015) Applied theatre: aesthetics. Bloomsbury Methuen Drama, London

Yakhforoshha A, Emami SAH, Mohammadi N, Cheraghi M, Mojtahedzadeh R, Mahmoodi-Bakhtiari B, Shirazi M (2017) Developing an integrated educational simulation model by considering art approach: teaching empathetic communication skills. Eur J Pers Cent Healthc 5(1):154–165

From Self-Centredness to Person-Centredness

5

Introduction

This chapter is the first of four which presents and discusses the main findings of the primary research conducted as part of my doctoral study. This part of the book seeks to present the results of a practical application through my primary research based on the conceptual framework as presented in Part 1. Each of the following four chapters is based on a main theme distilled through a process of analysis of the data collected from my doctoral study (Gale et al. 2013).

This chapter focuses on the first main theme, 'from self-centredness to person-centeredness'. This theme represents how the participants who took part in my study explored and challenged their perceived notion of self during the course. This theme follows the participants' journey from considering their sense of self through their attributes in what could be called a self-centred approach, towards a developed understanding of person-centredness and person-centred attributes. The use of the term self-centred here does not mean selfish, but rather a sense of self as individual, singular, and static, in many ways counter to the term person-centred. Participants reflected on how these self-centred approaches and attributes may relate to person-centred nursing. They then considered whether effective nursing requires a certain type of 'self' or whether an abstraction of self through 'selflessness' was more desirable.

The path of this chapter reflects the path taken by the participants in the drama workshops as part of my primary research. This began when the group reflected on aspects of the self and how a self might interrelate with others. This led to how the group understood the distinctiveness of person-centredness and person-centred nursing through experience and interaction. Towards the end of the sessions, the group developed a 'knowing self' which understood the criticality of self-awareness in being person-centred. After all, the self is a person. As it seems then, reflecting on the self and how the self relates to others is a crucial first step.

© The Author(s), under exclusive license to Springer Nature Switzerland AG 2024
K. Tizzard-Kleister, *Applied Drama and Person-Centred Nursing*, https://doi.org/10.1007/978-3-031-77208-5_5

Throughout Part 2 reference will be made to responses to the drama course through a series of related workshops that I designed and co-facilitated as part of my doctoral study. These are given as direct quotations. There are three different forms; text from the CPRs, text from my participant-observer journal, and text from the follow-up focus group interview. If given as the name of the participant, then the source is the individual CPR text. If it is given as 'focus group', then the quotation comes from the interview. Finally, if given as 'field notes', then this originates from my participant-observer journal.

Each of the chapters in Part 2 is structured around subheadings that serve as lightning rods to base the discussion around conceptually, but refer to the practice and experience involved with the drama course. Extracts of data are given to provide context to the discussion, to reinforce a point made, to seed statements and arguments, and to present the experience on the course in a more direct way than a purely abstract discussion. I jump and shift between descriptions of conceptual inference and pragmatic applications. I am resisting the urge to separate these aspects from each other, which may make for a clearer articulation of the results of my study, but remove the flow and process of reaching these points of new understanding. I hope, therefore, that Part 2 presents the findings of my study as a narrative, interconnected and contingent.

The Participants

Before this chapter begins in earnest, I want to present an overview of the people who volunteered to participate in my study. Below is a brief profile of each of the participants who volunteered to participate, provided consent, attended the course, and contributed to the data collected. The names below are used throughout the rest of Part 2. The names given here are pseudonyms to protect the identity of the participants, but the brief details about who they are give an insight into the people who took part. All of these participants were first-year nursing students at the time of the study, consented to participate, provide data, and for that data to be used in this study. The course consisted of a series of drama workshops totalling 24 h of face-to-face contact time. Each participant attended the majority of the sessions and provided data for the study. They were a joy to be around, full of insight and enthusiasm and each strove to be the best nurses that they could be.

Jamie—Jamie appears to be in her early to mid-20s and does not have previous experience working in care, or the performing arts. Jamie lives a short distance away, though stays in Derry/Londonderry during the week. She has a sister who now lives in Australia. They are very close, and Jamie professes that she misses her sister deeply.

Morgan—Morgan appears to be in her early to mid-twenties and has taken part in yoga and meditation classes before but does not seem to have experience in the performing arts. She attended the North West Regional College in Derry/Londonderry, which is next door to the Magee campus of Ulster University, where she studied Health and Care. After the first week and a half of the drama course, Morgan does not attend again. She has provided invaluable data for the study and has consented fully to it being used.

Nic—Nic appears to be in his early to late twenties and lives in Newry, which is a two-hour drive from Derry/Londonderry, but he seems to stay during the week. He works in a pub in Newry over the weekend alongside his studies. Nic does not have previous experience working in healthcare, or the performing arts.

Rowan—Rowan appears to be in her mid to late 20s and has two young children. She lives near Dungiven, her commute is reportedly a 45-min drive to/from Derry/Londonderry, and she often travels along with Gabrielle and Hannah. Rowan has taken some yoga classes before and has some experience working in healthcare, but no experience of the performing arts.

Alice—Alice appears to be in her late 20s to early 30s. She is a course rep for the first-year nursing cohort. Alice has experience in drama, having previously studied drama at university. Partway through my course Alice disclosed that at this other university, she experienced a traumatic incident. After disclosing this to me and the nursing staff liaison after a session, she is quick to assure us that she is finding engaging with the course a positive, safe, and almost therapeutic experience. Alice lives near Enniskillen which is an hour and a half drive from Derry/Londonderry, but seemingly stays in Derry/Londonderry during the week. She does not have previous experience working in healthcare.

Gabrielle—Gabrielle appears to be in her late 20s to early 30s, has two young children and lives near Dungiven. She and Rowan often travel together with Hannah. She cares for her grandmother who has dementia. Gabrielle visits her grandmother twice a week along with her family, replacing the care which was in place as she believes the care she and her family give is more personal and effective. Gabrielle does not have previous experience in professional healthcare or the performing arts.

Hannah—Hannah appears to be in her mid to late 20s. She struggles with weight bearing through one arm, as she reportedly broke a bone in her hand a few years ago, and it is still sore during and after extended weight bearing. Hannah has previous experience working as a healthcare assistant, but no experience of the performing arts. Hannah lives near Dungiven and travels with Gabrielle and Rowan.

The rest of this chapter will be presented in the same way as the following three comprising Part 2. The data from this study, including the responses from the participants which are given verbatim, will punctuate the discussion of ideas and practices that formed the study. I hope this part gives an insight into how drama can be practically applied to person-centred nursing, and how doing this in an interdisciplinary way from a conceptual to a practical level is challenging, yet incredibly rewarding. This part is where the rubber hits the road, where the ideas become reality and are subsequently analysed in context to the previous part and the wider context of the field of drama and nursing.

Reflecting on the Self, Understanding Inter-Relationality

The drama-based course provided opportunities for participants to open up and share aspects about themselves they might not have shared otherwise. Participants reflected on how they felt about themselves, including their traits and perceived weaknesses and how they used certain coping mechanisms in various situations. For example, participants displayed an ability to identify aspects of self-sabotage, which serve as barriers for them to care for others. Moreover, the group explored potential ways to address these barriers by adapting their perception of self to suit different situations as well as identifying features of their perceived selves which felt unchangeable.

> *I always use laughter as a nervous coping scheme. Now sometimes I can't tell when I laugh for enjoyment. I really enjoy my own space […] Sometimes I can show people who I am […] I have accepted that I am different.* (Hannah: 209–216)

The drama course encouraged the participants to try and take on different roles during exercises and SRPs. The participants discovered how they might practically take on these roles and how these different roles helped or hindered their interactions in different situations. The findings suggest that encouraging the use of multiple roles, particularly when exploring interactive situations in an educational context, aids participants in developing an understanding of how to perform a suitable role concerning the needs of others. This affirms the importance of relationality at the moment when considering the 'attributes' that 'help shape how we develop relationships', as McCormack & McCance suggest (2010: p. 56). I argue that the 'prerequisites' suggested in the PCNF are attributes that are recognised in a given moment rather than inherent virtues or unshakeable traits. Considering them in this way helps individuals to become person-centred nurses by adopting a constantly shifting and relational approach to understanding oneself and others.

A strong example of this was how participants expressed an appreciation of certain personal traits and abilities for their utility in building positive relationships with others. Meanwhile, they identified the value in traits such as kindness and actions such as listening to others in establishing these caring therapeutic relationships. This suggests that engaging in the course facilitated an openness that many participants took to willingly and generously. Notably, this openness began with ideas that are self-centred and trait-focused, but quickly through the notion of engaging with others developed into an appreciation for person-centred ideas.

> *I value my kindness that I display towards people and willingness to help.*
> *I value people's differences and I love to learn about different cultures and listening to stories.* (Jamie: 654–657)

The course directly engaged participants to feel the presence of others, advocating for contemplation and cooperation in creating a communally performed sympathetic presence. The participants' journey throughout the course reflects a move away from being focused on themselves in isolation to being more open to noticing aspects of others. This could in a broad sense be called the 'story' of the other person, their 'narrative identity' as McCormack and McCance (2010) put it. This led the participants to recognise how these stories relate to the perceptions they have of themselves and their own stories. Moreover, the participants understood how their presence is affected by how they actively and responsively present themselves and then how they are perceived by others. As such, the concept of presence became an important prism through which to present oneself and understand the presence of others, on the 'stage' of everyday life.

In performance and drama-based terms, stage presence is often stated to rely on 'forgetting' a sense of 'the self', whilst committing to the form of a given performance–as Umathum (2015: p. 111) amongst others has theorised. This deeply resonates with the findings of this study where being present as a nurse relies on moving from self-centred to person-centred concerns. Both drama and nursing, it seems, task the practitioner to lose themselves in the moment, to then find and relate to others in that moment and also with the moment itself. The drama course provided a space for both critical discourse and experience of this 'loss of self' but has gone further to infuse this 'loss' with an increased awareness of persons and personhood through directly embodying the role of others. This led to a deeper appreciation of the need to listen to the 'stories' that others share and the unique ways they articulate these stories. By embodying and performing these roles themselves they were allowed to, as Nolan (2009) puts it, test their 'powers of articulation against their limits of articulation' (p. 215).

This was made possible through both critical reflection and engaging with embodied knowledge. In discussing person-centred approaches to leadership Lynch (2015) states that 'engaging in critical discourse helps a person to reflect on the assumptions, beliefs and presuppositions they hold, and which constrain their view and perception of the world' (p. 6). Concurrently engaging in critical discourse influenced by the bodily experience provided by the drama exercises and SRPs, the participants were afforded an inner and outer view into the perspective of others. This was an active and embodied feeling. For the participants, this helped them to tap into an active state of sensation where notions of the self are suspended so that one might better feel and understand the feelings of others. This was most notable in the applied puppetry sessions and those who played the role of the puppeteer. In this role, the participants reportedly attuned to the feelings of the simulated patient as well as those playing family members and responded accordingly with believable actions in the role-play scenarios. This could be argued to be an articulation of what Titchen et al. (2017) discuss as '[e]mbodied knowledge', in their search for an ontological and epistemic framework for person-centred nursing (p. 37). For them this is a knowledge that 'may not reach conscious thought and so [might] not be verbalised' (Ibid), making it perhaps more difficult to include in traditional ontological or epistemological frameworks but vitally important in person-centred nursing. Beyond the difficulty of including embodied knowledge in existing nursing theories and frameworks, a distinct gap between theory and practice creates a further difficulty in creating and implementing embodied knowledge in nursing research, education, and ultimately into practice.

Though the notion of a gap between theory and practice has been explored before in applications of drama and nursing (Ekebergh et al. 2004) the distinction between technical skill acquisition and interpersonal skill acquisition is underexplored. This suggests that communication practices and general interactions in early-stage nursing education are often carried out on 'auto-pilot'. Furthermore, this suggests that responses and interactions are encouraged to be pre-programmed for student nurses, echoing the notion of Ritzer's (2004) 'McDoctors'. What is specifically lost in this mechanistic paradigm can be described as 'response-ability' (Haraway 2008; Hamera 2013). What the findings of this study tell us about this in particular is that it is not just the ability to respond spontaneously in the moment which is lost, but also the engagement and *responsibility* that one has when interacting with others. Throughout the course the participants developed their 'response-ability', suggesting they had a clearer understanding of the need for open and responsive interactions. This led to a deeper engagement with others, and a heightened sense of responsibility to engage with others as part of nursing work. The findings of this study strongly suggest a closer look at communication education and training to take this into account.

The course provided the group with moments to pause and reflect as well as opportunities to actualise their learning through these reflections. The group did not just consider aspects of their own identities, and how to potentially change them, they practiced and actualised these changes. This shows the development of skills in response-ability through practice and experience. Participants commented on the interactive experiences offered by the course leading to gaining knowledge and skills more effectively. Some participants expressed a heightened awareness of the validity of the knowledge others had as well as the value of learning through doing, particularly in contrast to didactic lecture-based learning.

> *Gabrielle: You can go into a lecture and spend two hours in a talk, and I'm like, oh my God. But like, listening to [senior nurses], or even that day we came in here listening to actual registered nurses saying how they would do it. You learn more –*
> *[talking over each other]*
> *Rowan: You learn more from the, like drama, like –*
> *Jamie: Yeah –*
> *Gabrielle: talking and doing rather than standing there reading off a board –*
> *Alice: Than a lecture.* (Focus group: 1444–1453)

Though it is clear that the group were experiencing an engaging new approach to learning, including learning through inter-relating with others around them, the purpose of this learning was also clear to them. The content of the course was delivered in experiential, interactive, and dialogical ways. This enhanced the group's understanding and practice of person-centredness as a key topic—particularly concerning their reflection on 'self' in relation to others.

Understanding Person-Centredness Through Experiential and Interactive Learning

The drama course evidenced the need for a different educational approach to communication than those employed for technical skill acquisition. Even within role plays without the involvement of technical tasks participants still seem somewhat fixated on achieving tasks technically and mechanistically. Arrighi et al. (2018) praise healthcare-based role play for 'its value for practising professional communication skills and building confidence for the real workplace' (99–100). However, in their study on the benefits of specialised actor training to enhance standardised patient performance in SRP they describe most role-play interactions as predominantly 'goal-driven' rather than 'situation-driven'. This is where the simulation focuses on achieving particular goals rather than exploring—and experiencing—the presented situation. This is particularly pertinent when role play leads to any type of formal engagement in which there are a series of outcomes for the participant to achieve, such as OSCE assessments. There is thus a tension between SRP designed to assess, and SRP designed as a learning process.

Participants highlight the lack of time for working nurses to notice the distinct identities of others. Instead of having time to notice and communicate in any meaningful way with patients, the participants observed how some nurses only felt able to rush through tasks to get their shift over as soon as possible. This shows how the participants demonstrated an ability to identify the issues facing a working nurse in terms of paying attention to and communicating with others, and in particular, the challenges facing person-centred nursing being put into practice.

> *Rowan: Definitely. There's* [sic] *some better than others obviously. There's* [sic] *really good ones.*
> *Karl: What do we think might be the reason that they're not noticing these things?*
> *Rowan: They're just getting their job done.*
> *Alice: Lack of communication. With the patient*
> *[general agreement]*
> *Gabrielle: Some are there so long, or are just in and out.*
> *Rowan: They're there to pass the day, just to get the day ended, get the day out, get the money and go home.* (Focus group: 1213–1222)

Also apparent was the depth and awareness of knowledge transmission between peers. For the participants, it appeared that the activities, discussions, and reflections in the course highlighted how we interactively learn not just information but value systems, emotional management, practical communication skills, and much more from those around us. For example, Hannah reflected on her peers' performance in role plays, identifying the types of traits within these performances that she felt were valuable. This demonstrates an attentiveness to the traits displayed by others to address the given circumstance of that particular moment and a recognition of the value that you place on these as an individual. This practice also promotes an active positive regard, resonating with Roger's notion of unconditional positive regard as a cornerstone of person-centred practice (Rogers 1961).

I value Rowan's passion for her family member [...] I valued Nic's communication skills during our role-play. [...] I valued Nic's approach to planning the task. (Hannah: 595–599)

The interactive approach afforded by the dramatic practices contributed to, and sustained, a developed level of trust and cooperation amongst the participants. This allowed the group to address difficult content in interactive ways which included emotional expression, self-exploration, discussing perceptions of others, and more in front of and between participants. The group began to show an understanding that person-centredness relies not on personal traits, but on relationships, and even began to experience the potential learning, self-realisation, and joy to be gained by engaging in emotional and trusting relationships. The course seemed to develop a sense of resilience by highlighting the benefits of deep acting and emotional engagement, avoiding emotional dissonance (Delgado et al. 2017). In this way, the course facilitated a congenial space (White 2009). This was seen, for example, in an exercise tasking the participants to close their eyes and imagine themselves in various situations, culminating in what they felt was a safe space, and how the group shared what these safe spaces were to them, and in some cases, this was emotionally challenging for the participants to do.

This exercise elicited powerful responses as the group talked about these safe spaces and the things that constituted these imagined spaces for them. For instance, Jamie commented on imagining a framed photograph of her sister who now lives away from home. She found thinking about her sister, whom she missed deeply, very emotional. Rather than hiding this or asking to stop she openly shared her feelings with the group. The whole group could not help but be moved by this. Afterwards, it was observable that though crying, Jamie appeared and reported being content, suggesting an emotional openness, respect, and trust between her and the group. Jamie demonstrated an ability to tackle this emotional dilemma in the space, which for her at that moment was a dilemmatic space in the context of not having her sister nearby anymore (Preston 2016). Her trust in those around her meant this dilemma was addressed openly and with the support of the group. This showed the potential for taking part in this space in the drama course to be in these difficult spaces whilst feeling comforted. In these moments the drama course provided a space of potentiality in which to share and support each other through infusing a congenial space with the inevitable dilemmatic ones (White 2009; Preston 2016; Sloan 2018).

We ask if Jamie is OK and give her some time. Jamie says she is fine, I do not believe this is emotional distress, but a display of emotion which would only occur in this safe space alongside trusted co-participants. (Field notes: 1801–1804)

Crucially this was not a personal story that was sought by us but *offered generously*. As many applied drama theorists argue, seeking stories from participants that are then re-told and re-staged for some dramatic purpose can be a questionable approach (Thompson 2009; Sloan 2018). This is doubly so for difficult stories, especially when done in an insensitive way. A significant part of the skill and art of applied drama facilitation can be said to be recognising when participants find activities challenging, and providing suitable support and responses to that need to help that person participate in the way they wish to (Preston 2016; Hepplewhite 2020). It can be said that giving Jamie time and space in that moment is crucial for creating a space of potentiality, as she navigates the tricky circumstance of the dilemma she is grappling with, whilst leaning into the congeniality of the space we had all created together. So often moments like these are either avoided or brushed over—or on the other end of the spectrum given too much attention. The drama course and the exercises we explored made this a moment to linger in, to privilege, and to validate—but not to stultify within. Not feeling as though sharing how you feel, what is really on your mind, can easily lead to distress, just as being coerced to share can. This process is a constant balance of personal needs, highlighting how the concepts and practices of applied drama facilitation are extremely resonant with those from PCN. Jamie's moment of vulnerability created a brave space, a space where we are invited to respond with compassion. This indicates how emotions and feelings can be shared amongst a group, and distress can be avoided (or rather embraced) by mutual respect and sympathetic presence in a group of peers. Sympathetic presence, therefore, offers the applied drama facilitator an approach to engage with participants, to attend to their feelings and personhood, and to support them with an engaged presence.

Drama also offers a space to address and at times share emotions and dilemmas acting within oneself. There were many moments—informed by the participants' personal experiences of care work as well as their nursing studies—where traditional roles in healthcare environments were explored and challenged. The strong working relationships helped the group to share experiences which served as valuable teaching and learning points. This revealed, for instance, how difficult it is to interact with patients who do not act as you would like, or that a nurse is not immune from the suffering of those they care for.

Through this discussion Hannah, Rowan and Gabrielle express stories involving patients with challenging behaviours, which run contrary to this normalised idea that the traditional notion of patient is of suffering - a nurse may suffer too. (Field notes: 1964–1968)

Through engaging in the drama course, the participants explored and understood personhood in practical terms. They expressed an understanding of personhood as a relational expression of self which is in constant dialogue with other selves. This supports the suggestions of existing PCN researchers such as McCormack and McCance (2010), Lieshout and Cardiff (2015), and Dewing et al. (2017). Dewing et al. (2017) specifically draw attention to how Kitwood argues that 'personhood is absolute' as well as 'a social status awarded by another or others' (p. 24). In an attempt to light a path towards person-centred approaches to health research, Dewing et al. (2017) advocate for the inclusion of the multiple worldviews of those involved with the research. They suggest that Kitwood's definition inherently implies exclusion. As both a research project and pedagogy my study has included multiple worldviews in line with Dewing et al's thinking.

There is some noticeable success in how the design of the course allowed for open and person-centred research. Notably in the creative personal reflections which gave participants the freedom to reflect creatively, both without judgement on the content, or the perceived aesthetic quality of the reflection. I suggest that the drama-based approach supported a person-centred research environment and pedagogic space, which in turn helped the participants to directly experience a shift from self-focused thinking into person-centred ones. In these spaces, taking risks did not feel dangerous. Meanwhile, being vulnerable was a way to offer, and often receive, generosity and engagement from others through sympathetic presence. Moreover, in a practical sense, the participants saw that by approaching an understanding of— or at least engaging with and attending more closely to—the personhood of others and oneself it became easier to interact effectively in that given moment. Simply, the more you know yourself and the more you know others and are aware of the distinctions between yourself and that other, you can find easier ways to interact.

Particularly evident were reflections on how some participants felt that nurses should step back from their concerns and disregard their own needs to put a patient's needs first. Being aware of and considering the perspective of the patient—especially patients who are 'annoying'—was described as vital for a nurse to adjust their thinking and provide care. Participants therefore expressed an understanding of the need to and effect of adapting your presented self in nursing practice. Participants began displaying an awareness that people are distinct, and these people and their actions may affect you in certain ways. Moreover, they explore that each person might need to be met with an adapted presentation of self, requiring a shift from an idea of a static self to one that acknowledges and serves multiple selves. A few concepts here are sure to raise eyebrows. However, this is an indication of the beginnings of a journey to person-centredness. This represents a moment of spark, that though might not be exactly what we might want to teach and promote as a person-centred practice (IE, that a nurse's needs should be entirely disregarded in favour of a patient's needs), it indicates an awareness of the distinction between one's needs and the needs of others. They are expressing the understanding that to care for others, you need to be aware of what they need rather than assume it. Moreover, they demonstrate an understanding that others are driven by their needs, which affects how they interact with you.

By seeing how one's actions produce intersubjective meaning in an interaction, participants moved away from labelling people through their behaviour or emotions and recognised the potential harm in this. By applying ideas from Stanislavski's MoPA as described in Part 1, the group saw, for instance, how someone might appear angry, but that does not necessarily mean they are an angry person. Using actions provides a learning point into communication through inter-subjectivity, and how what someone does to another person strikes at the heart of interpersonal skills. One might appear angry, but they may be questioning you, for instance. These are understood to be constructed through difference, as participants begin to perceive others from their distinct personhood rather than assuming it.

As a nurse your problems should be left at the door no matter if you work in a hospital or community setting. Putting the patient's needs first. A nurse should never label a patient being [sic] *annoying or complaining, but they should take a step back and imagine what it would feel like to be in their shoes and adjust to the different changes, different patients* [sic]. (Gabrielle: 106–111)

Observationally, the participants demonstrated that the acting techniques being applied to the scenarios provided a framework to discuss how to interact differently and more effectively in situations which may be difficult to pre-empt. It also tasked participants to try performing different 'selves' by performing as different characters. Seen in particular in the early role-play tasks, where participants were given simple characters like 'nurse', 'patient' or 'family member', with simple objectives such as 'support family member' or 'disclose information'. These exercises were improvised, with feedback given to change the situation and provide participants with a different perspective on what they could do in the role-play through, for instance, performing 'actions' like 'to accuse', to achieve their objective.

The scene plays again, with Nic in particular taking more of a role in supporting everyone, and Hannah presenting more accountability. Rowan does well to continue accusing, which again knocks the others from their actions into providing information and "avoiding", prompting more argument. (Field notes: 1697–1702)

What became clear to the participants was that the drama-based course did not aim to explicitly teach them exactly what to do in a certain situation but focused on developing responsiveness, attentiveness, and spontaneity to better deal with a variety of situations. This lends credence to Lieshout and Cardiff's (2015) argument that the processes of PCN are not 'sequential steps', but a 'constant listening to self, others and context so that appropriate and intentional action can be undertaken' (p. 9). The group realised that though a caring exchange needed to be improvised, it could still be 'rehearsed' through the skills we explored. Hamington (2020) suggests that we are all capable of care, but most do not develop skills to reach their potential. As the participants expressed at the beginning of the drama course, the interactions which were explored were not entirely new to them and definitely within their capabilities to navigate. In this way, the dramatic performances served as a learning method towards purposeful action and interaction. The group realised one cannot prepare for every encounter. Instead one must prepare 'an architecture of caring skills including physical, emotional and intellectual habits' not just useful for the 'performance of care but also [influencing] who I am and how I subsequently address others' (Ibid: p. 33). This resonates with the notion of 'prerequisites' for nurses approaching PCN explained in the PCNF and taps into how we might understand and attend to others through a metaphorical translation (Tizzard-Kleister and Jennings 2020) of their perspective.

This is reflected in many instances when the participants reportedly felt sympathetic presence most. These were moments when the group worked together to create an ephemeral feeling of sympathetic presence throughout the environment at that given moment. As McCormack et al highlighted in 2015 in their retrospective of the state of PCN across the globe, 'health and social care cultures still need to evolve further so that they truly place people at the centre of their care in order to achieve effective and meaningful outcomes' (p. 3). I suggest that this drama-based model could serve as an educational method to begin to address creating and sustaining culture change through fostering relationships and helping groups to create and feel a communal sympathetic presence. The drama course as part of my doctoral study achieved this by teaching a relationship-based and person-centred approach to care through a performative approach to sympathetic presence, thereby aiming towards creating and sustaining person-centred environments and cultures from a grass-roots level. Person-centred researchers call for nurses who lead through action, citing this ability as a crucial role for future person-centred nurses to incite and sustain culture change (Lynch 2015; Eide and Cardiff 2017). Using drama within PCN education is an action-focused method which promotes an individual's agency and subsequently their ability to change culturally ingrained approaches—at least on an individual and small group level.

Participants in my study seemed to use and draw from the drama-based techniques to adapt and enhance their role-play scenarios. These activities helped the group see how important it is to be aware of how you communicate with others, as well as how easy this is to overlook, particularly when you are focused on yourself, or a clinical task. It was evident that this experience aided the participants' understanding of the uniqueness of each encounter with others. This appeared to lead to a recognition of the necessity to adapt how they presented themselves to both enhance the interaction and to suit the needs of those in their care as well as their own. This was understood to not mean an assumption of another's needs but as an interpretation of what that person presents there and then. This demonstrated a move away from self-centred considerations of how they felt able, or wanted, to interact, towards interacting with the distinct personhood of the person they interacted with at the forefront of their concerns.

> Rowan: *it's just the way that you could neglect your communication to people, not that you are acting [...], but if you're speaking to like a child you'd speak in an even tone, or if you're speaking to an adult then [pauses, possibly can't think of an example] stuff like that. So like, it's not acting, but it's...[tails off, possibly she can't find the right word to describe what she means].* (Focus Group: 128–131)

Though the participants were better able to identify their own and others' objectives within a given moment or a specific interaction, more could have been done to explore the idea of a Stanislavkian 'super-objective' (Stanislavski 1990). In actor training, this is where an actor tries to discover what their character wants and needs over a longer timeframe. A super-objective is often akin to a life goal. There is untapped potential to explore each participant's super objective as a nurse and as a person. Though they did not explore their super objectives, the participants reflected on the wider issues facing nurses. For instance, the group reflected on the difficulties facing those wishing to train to become nurses as well as the difficulties faced by staff in the practice of nursing, including a lack of time to be open and generous in self-reflection. For example, they pinpointed a lack of opportunity to pause, think and reflect during their work as a key difficulty pervading the work of nursing.

Jamie: Oh yes! I was just gunna say that the nurses probably don't just pause, you know sometimes–
Rowan: to think about things. (Focus group: 1332–1334)

This sense of a need to achieve a specific goal without taking pause or reflection was observable in early exercises and role plays. For instance, when interacting in role plays the participants who performed as an attending nurse initially focused on ensuring the correct use of terminology and delivering as much information as possible to their patients. This approach deviated from person-centredness, as the person became secondary to the aim of completing the technical or clinical task. I argue that in healthcare education SRP has been used more often as a way to assess competence, and not as a progressive and interactive learning method (Arrighi et al. 2018; Taylor et al. 2021). I argue further that the insight and expertise that drama professionals, educators, and theorists could bring to SRP has been overlooked. By discussing the SRPs with the participants using the approaches and terminology from applied drama and actor training, the participants could apply their new comprehension into practice and begin to be more comfortable with keeping the person, and the effect that their interactions had on them, as their focus.

Neilson and Reeves (2019) explore how using forum theatre, and other Boalian techniques, might help nursing students dealing with emotional communication in palliative care. Similarly to Neilson and Reeves' (2019) intervention, the aim of my drama course was not to assess the participants' communication skills empirically, but to explore, develop, challenge and extend 'their perception of their ability to communicate' (p. 11). This included shifting the participant's perception of communication in nursing from auxiliary to ancillary work as well as interlinking good communication with the effective completion of technical procedures, as well as more person-centred outcomes. Considering the findings of this study, I suggest that re-considering not just the balance between soft and technical skills, but the approach with which they are taught, practiced, and applied is vitally important to ensuring consistent person-centred communication. It is asserted that the pedagogic methodology used in my drama course could potentially be the first step to building a technical and easily usable approach to developing effective and interactive 'soft' skills. Moreover, I assert that weaving this approach amongst the education of clinical skills reinforces that both skill sets are necessary for competent person-centred nurses.

The variety and adaptability in the types of scenarios explored in my course aided participants in recognising the uniqueness of every interaction. Meanwhile, the use of acting in the moment rather than over-preparing a set 'method' for dealing with each person further illustrated a move away from considering self as static to seeing self as constructed fluidly and in the moment of each different interaction. The use of terminology like 'character' and 'acting' from drama-based activities gave the group a specific language to discuss these issues concretely. Although they maintained a wariness with applying these words to others, such as patients, perhaps for fear of minimising their lives by calling it an 'act'. The group were quick to make it clear that real patients are not acting yet using acting skills may help the participants interact with them.

> Rowan: as you said, when you are acting it, I was able to act to you as a bad family member.
> Hannah: yeah you were brilliant
> [laughter all around]
> Rowan: when sometimes that is the case, and you know - they're not acting.
> Jamie: Uhuh, that's it yeah. You just don't know what you're-
> Rowan: what buttons you press to somebody –
> Gabrielle: or how different each day is.
> Jamie: I know, so many different characters.
> Rowan: oh so many of them, that's right. (Focus group: 2000–2010)

This demonstrated an understanding that though not real, the dramatic practices related to real situations and that taking part in dramatic practice helps understand real situations. On a conceptual level, the participants understood that the 'real' and the 'not-real' can co-relate in an educational space to produce active learning about others and oneself. However, more exploration could be made of the wariness to see how others 'act', indicating that this course may have been weighed too heavily on personal exploration of the 'self', rather than using similar techniques to recognise important aspects of others. Perhaps ironically, this is often highlighted as a key outcome for drama-based approaches in nurse education (Arveklev et al. 2018; Mermikides 2020; Kyle et al. 2023). I am not suggesting that this is not an evident outcome of my study, simply that this aspect was expected to be identified more than it was. I speculate that this may be due to the design of the study, which included more weighting on 'skills' development than applications to SRP. Furthermore, I envisage that if this approach was applied to first-year nursing education, it would seed students' studies, and we may see a development of how they apply these skills to their SRPs and practice over the following years of their studies. In hindsight, a follow-up study with my participant cohort throughout their studies would have provided invaluable longitudinal data on the retention of these approaches, and explore how the participants could apply theory into practice throughout their studies in comparison to their peers.

Participants expressed a deeper understanding of nursing concepts relating to the self in the presence of others, as well as the PCNF. It seemed that looking at the PCNF through physical activities with others aided how some participants understood it. The participants could see how their performance in the role of a person-centred nurse hinged on an ability to recognise and attend to the authentically presented aspects of another's personhood in a facilitative way. This finding gives weight to Lieshout and Cardiff's (2015) assertion that 'being attentive to the personhood of others and self, embedded within complex and dynamic contexts' is a key part of being a person-centred nurse, or as they prefer—facilitator (p. 8). This dramatically shifted the participants' perceptions of the role the person-centred nurse has in a caring exchange and subsequently how they should present themselves to others. Participants began to see their role as a person-centred nurse differently.

Looking at the person-centred framework in pieces of work helped me understand the framework on a deeper level. (Alice: 917–918)

In many instances, a key first step on the journey to this deeper level of awareness seemed to be an enhanced 'knowing self', and a recognition of how the self is a person within an interaction. More precisely, it is understanding the effect the self has on both the person you are and how you relate to the personhood of others through this self.

The Self Is a Person Too, How a 'Knowing Self' Enhances Person-Centredness

Many exercises and activities in the course highlighted for the participants how easy it is to overlook how they communicate with others. As it is for many other student nurses, the participants assumed their ability to communicate to be broadly positive and effective. It could be that many nursing students have spent little to no time reflecting on their ability to communicate, let alone developing a practice to explore and improve their communication skills. On a broad level, there seem to be scant frames of reference for students to measure against what makes one a 'good' communicator, other than comparisons to individuals they see as role models. During and after the course, the participants displayed an increased awareness of communication as a skill, more pointedly they gained a finer ability to identify good practice from bad practice. Intriguingly, and perhaps running counter to the generally held perception in nursing education and practice, the group discovered that these skills are difficult and, just like technical skills, they need practice. I argue that using drama in nursing education could offer two key things; a frame of reference for good communication through demonstration and role play and a framework for analysing and improving communication.

Some very specific areas and applications of interactive skills arose in the course. The notions of embodiment and cognitive function, relating to issues like dementia, a patient receiving a bad diagnosis, unresponsive patients and more, were raised and discussed in the context of presence. Participants expressed a deeper understanding of the distinctness of every individual's personhood in relation to their unique needs, suggesting a developed appreciation of personhood conceptually and practically through the activities. Participants appreciated that not every person needs the same type of interaction. In the majority of cases, the group explored how the presence of the other and what this tells you about them provides an insight into the appropriate presence of the nurse in response to the situation. This is a crucial place to begin a sympathetic interaction. This seemed to highlight to the participants that the experiences of the nurse are not as important at this moment as the other's feelings and needs, displaying a distinct move from self-centred concerns to person-centred interactions.

Hannah: it's more than your verbals when you're being sympathetic

> *Rowan: [slightly over-the-top of Hannah] it's not just talking to someone*
> *Gabrielle: if somebody is having, for example somebody had a really bad diagnosis and*
> *she didn't want anything, she just wanted somebody there.*
> *Rowan: it's just your presence.*
> *Gabrielle: it's the way you approach them*
> *[general agreement]*
> *[...]*
> *Jamie: yeah.*
> *Rowan: maybe your presence is enough for somebody.*
> *Jamie: yeah, you don't necessarily have to have gone through yourself.*
> *Gabrielle: it's more about them going through it.*
> *Jamie: yeah* (Focus Group: 367–382)

This revelation that often presence is enough was reciprocated and agreed upon by many of the participants. Sympathetic presence thus moves away from passivity and seeks to encourage action and engagement alongside emotional attunement. This finding evidences that notion and adds that sympathetic presence is a communicative process. However, the participants discovered that communication can be deeply affected by the status and power of those who are interacting. They explored this through role plays and specific activities alongside negotiating the difficulties a person-centred nurse might encounter in interactions with others. For instance, when a nurse cares for others these others can often be described as dependent on them. This presents difficulties in communicating in a person-centred way that emphasises making shared decisions as a key person-centred process. As the participants explored it is easy to dismiss, assume or control the care given to a person when they are dependent on you. Simplican (2015) challenges how Kittay emphasises 'permanent vulnerability' as a key characteristic of dependency (Simplican 2015: p. 19). Simplican presents an alternative by drawing on person-centred planning and suggests the notion of 'complex dependency', where dependents and those caring for them are both vulnerable, meanwhile they are also both capable of causing harm to the other (Ibid). The notion of complex dependency helps to shine a light on how difficult it can be for both parties to communicate effectively across what is a traditionally imbalanced power relationship between carer and care receiver. This is pertinent for person-centred approaches which advocate for centralising the person in healthcare.

These power imbalances provided the basis for some of the most interesting simulated encounters in the drama course, engaging the participants in the task of navigating these situations in a variety of ways. The findings of this study suggest that drama-based approaches offer a way to attune to the desires and needs of others through closer attention and understanding of the huge variety of meanings in their self-expression. As a result, this expands one's understanding of one's communicative potential. Simplican states that when caring for others with 'profound mental impairments' carers must 'decipher the person's unspoken interests, desires, and projects' whilst distinguishing 'the desires of their charge from their own' (2015: p. 220). Though this is stated in the context of a power and status relationship between someone with and someone without mental impairments, the thrust of this argument is far more universal than one may think, particularly considering Calvert's

(2020) notion of 'debility' as a universal human condition. Importantly, the findings of this study confirm that drama approaches and PCN not only enhance communication with those who have profound and 'easily identifiable' needs but may also be infused into communication as an everyday practice with all people, particularly in a care context. It is thus an essential part of performing sympathetic presence and being a person-centred nurse.

This extended into occurrences where participants developed an understanding of the distinctions between their personhood and the personhood of others, and an ability to work through these differences. The group explored and articulated how presence might be felt and then communicated by a nursing practitioner or a patient. Participants were able to identify how their presence may affect how others perceive them, and the importance of using their bodies and presence to communicate to others, suggesting the participants understood how personhood could be embodied through presence. Nic even expressed this understanding on an abstract and imagined level, identifying situations where this may be keenly felt by a person.

Nic: I think if a person is tending to be walking fast and running about the place you don't feel like any sympathy is being shown to me if I was a patient, it was a nurse or doctor running about the place frantically trying to get A B C D E done, you don't feel like, okay I'm being looked at properly here. (Focus Group: 605–609)

Interacting with mannequins showed the participants how a patient and their feelings could be easily overlooked by heightening the 'object-ness' of that patient, pointing towards the difficulty in communicating sensitively between two people (or puppets) who are greatly different. Jacobs et al. (2017) make the point that using technology in healthcare brings us face-to-face with existing issues revolving around how a practitioner takes or gives control in 'order for the person to use one's voice and capacities for self-determination' (p. 65). The use of applied puppetry brings this tension from both a research and practical perspective into stark contrast, whilst resisting the drive for technologically advanced, automated, mannequins. Using puppetry brings an object towards the human *through an application of the human*, and is deeply interested in the notion of giving or taking the power of self-determination.

Instead of being focused on bestowing personhood onto others or directly controlling a patient's journey from illness to health, the participants began to consider the role of the person-centred nurse as more closely aligned to recognising and remaining open to the distinctly different perspectives of others and subsequently to help them to achieve their needs in collaboration. This role, as Lieshout and Cardiff (2015) suggest, is closely tied to the role of a facilitator. Drawing from Preston's (2016) work on applied drama and facilitation, this idea should extend to 'critical facilitation'. The participants could see how their work as person-centred nurses 'is done *relationally* - in context, between people, and against a socio-political background', just as Preston describes the work of critical facilitators (2016: p. 17).

The group learnt that their personhood might influence how they approached performing that role. For instance, in the drama course, the participants actively adopted different performed roles for the sake of the simulations and exercises. Some of these roles were more or less comfortable to the participants. For example, during the 'killer queen' exercise[1] some relished the power they had over others when given the role of queen whilst others struggled with wielding the absolute authority implied in the role as it did not align with their perceived personhood. However, armed with this enhanced perception of themselves they were able to adapt their approach. As such, the findings of my study suggest that to understand personhood in practice is to be more attuned and attentive to the feelings and preferences of others, as well as our own, in that given moment.

Participants expressed an understanding of the unique needs of their patients in different situations. Resonant to Hepplewhite's (2020) notion, the group reported an 'attunement' to the needs of others. In this case, this attunement was specifically from the other's perspective rather than the perspective of their carer, they also displayed the ability to adapt their presence to suit this, including through non-verbal exchanges. In one particularly striking instance, Gabrielle described how she applied her understanding of personhood as embodied and relying on co-presence which she had developed through the drama course in her practice learning. In this instance, she acted differently than her colleagues, mostly fully registered nurses, by being more present towards a non-verbal and non-mobile patient. This was a display of a performed and aesthetic gesture, which afforded Gabrielle and her patient agency and reaffirmed the need for embodied and interactive affect to actualise care (Nolan 2009; Thompson 2023; Prentki 2023). Specifically, Gabrielle ensured that she spoke to this patient, and used her body language to express being present to them, even if they did not show an obvious response. Reportedly, Gabrielle put these concepts into practice almost exclusively through the notion of being present and using presence to communicate sympathy and care.

> Gabrielle: It's something nobody else did.
>   Karl: Did anything within the drama course help with that?
>   Gabrielle: Uh, probably something more with the [...] presence than anything, like [they] knew you were there, I think [they] genuinely knew what you were saying – (Focus group: 1239–1243)

In the case of this research study, the task of creating and maintaining person-centred workplaces and/or educational environments permeated with sympathetic presence is both personal *and* political. As evidenced by this study, drama-based approaches teach student nurses to be aware of their agency and to practice ways in which to use this agency in positive ways, whilst continually maintaining a focus on all the people involved in each experience and system. In this context, this

---

[1] Where one person is given an extreme high status as the queen/king, everyone else is given the lowest status imaginable. This is articulated in that the queen/king could "kill" them with a clap of their hands or click of their fingers. The game involves improvising around that situation, exploring how our behaviours change when in an extremely unbalanced power dynamic. We playfully changed the role of queen/king to "ward manager", bringing the situation closer to the lived experience of the participants.

interdisciplinary methodology goes beyond what drama and health pioneer Mike White envisaged as how the arts might contribute to 'maintaining and enhancing a culture of person-centred care', as 'an important *adjunct* to health services' (White 2009: p. 121; emphasis added). Instead, the implication from the findings of this research study is that there is huge potential for this approach to go beyond an *adjunct* and to be applied and *integrated* into person-centred nursing pedagogy and healthcare training more interconnectedly. This aligns the approach with what Preston (2016) extols, that the most effective applied drama interventions are those 'embedded into […] working structures' (p. 42). This goes beyond shorter-term drama interventions to help students with role play assessments, towards giving them time and space, opportunity, and institutional support to begin to fully embody the role of the person-centred nursing practitioner. It moves SRP from being 'goal-focused' to 'scenario-focused' (Arrighi et al. 2018). As interacting with others is a crucial aspect of PCN, and sympathetic presence is the main process through which to do that, these skills are essential for PCN education. What drama has been evidenced to provide for PCN education here is an approach to build an enhanced 'knowing self' in practitioners, and a greater outward awareness towards others. In short, a practical way to develop an understanding of personhood.

Actor training through the MoPA in particular promoted participant's abilities to overcome personal vulnerabilities in interactions and helped better perform effective caring roles. In the early attempts at SRP, and some other drama-based exercises, when the participants were tasked with adopting a 'character' it was difficult for them to see beyond their concerns and vulnerabilities. Particularly relevant was an observable and reported increase in anxiety when performing as an attending nurse. It could be argued that as early first-year students, the participants felt less confident with the knowledge involved in performing the role of a nurse. This could be extended to suggest that a focus on these, and other 'self-focused', concerns was the dominant factor in how engaged a participant could be in a SRP, as well as the perceived need to present an authentic or genuine self.

As Macneill et al. (2014) note in their project following healthcare workers taking part in drama workshops, the intervention made it clear for the healthcare workers that during their work their 'emotional expression (but not necessarily their emotional feeling) needs to be appropriate to the role they are playing' (p. 52). This soon became clear to the participants of my drama course as well. Eventually, it seemed that the group were better able to recognise and address vulnerable feelings which created fear and anxiety in the first place. As a result, the group displayed an ability to pay more attention to others and, borrowing the language of the first main theme of this study, to move from selfhood to personhood.

It seems that actor training in particular was effective in helping the participants untangle the multitude of possibilities in their presented roles, which had the added effect of reducing the perceived anxiety in performing these roles. Moreover, I contend that this research study confirms the suggestion made by Macneill et al. (2014) that actor training taught in a committed fashion to healthcare workers offers a 'craft' to move beyond concepts of the authenticity of genuine presentations of self in favour of a relational and action-based approach to 'interacting sensitively and effectively with others' (p. 54). As a result, instead of focusing on feelings of personal anxiety or vulnerability—possibly due to feeling the pressure to present oneself as genuine or authentic—participants were better able to remain present in a given situation to notice the moods, desires, and needs of those around them—including themselves.

Conclusion

This chapter has explored the first main theme of my research study and illustrated how the group who took part in my drama course developed from an understanding of self-centeredness to one of person-centeredness. This chapter highlighted how drama promoted the notion that the role of the effective person-centred nurse should not be trait-based or individualistically focused but fluid and relational. For instance, the participants showed how their 'knowing self' was never static. More so, they learnt that a static 'knowing self' restricts growth and learning, whilst making interacting with others difficult.

Through engaging with the course, participants gained a greater awareness of the concept of personhood and how it relates to fluid identity and relational processes, as opposed to attribute-focused notions of a static self. The participants reached this learning experientially and interactively, engaging their minds and bodies in unison to develop practical methods drawn from drama-based techniques to embody and respect the embodiment of personhood in a caring exchange. This theme therefore reflects the steps taken by the group from thinking through self-centredness to thinking through person-centredness. The chapter has also highlighted how this exploration of self could be extended by further application of Stanislavki's concept of the super-objective, supporting students to develop a robust perspective of their beliefs and values and seeing this as an important aspect of PCN.

The process of moving from self-centred to person-centred served as a partner and precursor to the phenomenon associated with the next theme: overcoming vulnerability. The next chapter will explore that theme in depth.

References

Arrighi G, Irvine C, Joyce B, Kristi Haracz K (2018) Reimagining 'role' and 'character': an approach to acting training for role-play simulation in the tertiary education setting. Appl Theatre Res 6(2):89–106

Arveklev SH, Berg L, Wigert H, Morrison-Helme M, Lepp M (2018) Nursing students experiences of learning about nursing through drama. Nurse Educ Pract 28:60–65

Calvert D (2020) Convivial theatre: care and debility in collaborations between non-disabled and learning disabled theatre makers. In: Stuart Fisher A, Thompson J (eds) Performing care: new perspectives on socially engaged performance. Manchester University Press, Manchester, pp 85–102

Delgado C, Upton D, Ranse K, Furness T, Foster K (2017) Nurses' resilience and the emotional labour of nursing work: an integrative review of empirical literature. Int J Nurs Stud 70:71–88

Dewing J, Eide T, McCormack B (2017) Philosophical perspectives on person-centredness for healthcare research. In: McCormack B, Dulmen S, Eide H, Skovdahl K, Eide T (eds) Person-centred nursing research. Wiley Blackwell, Chichester, pp 19–30

Eide T, Cardiff S (2017) Leadership research: a person-Centred agenda. In: McCormack B, Dulmen S, Eide H, Skovdahl K (eds) Person-centred healthcare research. Wiley-Blackwell, Chichester, pp 95–116

Ekebergh M, Lepp M, Dahlberg K (2004) Reflective learning with Drama in nursing education—a Swedish attempt to overcome the theory praxis gap. Nurse Educ Today 24:622–628

Gale N, Heath G, Cameron E, Rashid S, Redwood S (2013) Using the framework method for the analysis of qualitative data in multi-disciplinary health research. BMC Med Res Methodol 13:117. [Online] Available from: https://bmcmedresmethodol.biomedcentral.com/articles/10.1186/1471-2288-13-117. Accessed 9 Feb 2018

Hamera J (2013) Response-ability, vulnerability, and other(s') bodies. In: Johnson EP (ed) Cultural struggles: performance, ethnography, praxis. University of Michigan Press, Ann Arbor, pp 306–310

Hamington M (2020) Care ethics and improvisation: can performance care? In: Stuart Fisher A, Thompson J (eds) Performing care: new perspectives on socially engaged performance. Manchester University Press, Manchester, pp 21–35

Haraway D (2008) When species meet. University of Minnesota Press, Minneapolis

Hepplewhite K (2020) The applied theatre artist: responsivity and expertise in practice. Palgrave Macmillan, London

Jacobs G, van der Zijpp T, Lieshout F, van Dulmen S (2017) Research into person-centred healthcare technology: a plea for considering humanisation dimensions. In: McCormack B, Dulmen S, Eide H, Skovdahl K (eds) Person-Centred healthcare research. Wiley-Blackwell, Chichester, pp 61–68

Kyle R, Bastow F, Harper-McDonald B, Jeram T, Zahid Z, Nizamuddin M, Mahoney C (2023) Effects of student-led drama on nursing students' attitudes to interprofessional working and nursing advocacy: a pre-test post-test educational intervention study. Nurse Educ Today 123:1–11

Lieshout F, Cardiff S (2015) Reflections on being and becoming a person-centred facilitator. Int Pract Dev J 5. Available: https://www.fons.org/library/journal/volume5-person-centredness-suppl/article4. Accessed 9 Mar 2018

Lynch B (2015) Partnering for performance in situational leadership: a person-centred leadership approach. Int Pract Dev J 5. Available: https://www.fons.org/library/journal/volume5-person-centredness-suppl/article5. Accessed 13 Mar 2018

Macneill P, Gilmer J, Samarasekera DD, Hoon TC (2014) Actor training for doctors and other healthcare practitioners: a rationale from an actor's perspective. Glob J Arts Educ 4(2):49–55

McCormack B, McCance T (2010) Person-centred nursing: theory and practice. Wiley-Blackwell, Chichester

McCormack B, Borg M, Cardiff S, Dewing J, Jacobs G, Janes N, Karlsson B, McCance T, Mekki T, Porock D, Lieshout F, Wilson V (2015) Person-centredness—the 'state' of the art. Int Pract Dev J 5(1):1–15

Mermikides A (2020) Performance, medicine and the human. Methuen Drama, London

Neilson SJ, Reeves A (2019) The use of a theatre workshop in developing effective communication in paediatric end of life care. Nurse Educ Pract 36:7–12

Nolan C (2009) Agency and embodiment: performing gestures/producing cultures. Harvard University Press, Harvard

Prentki T (2023) A short essay on empathy, drama, and a new curriculum. Res Drama Educ 28(3):387–391

Preston S (2016) Applied theatre: facilitation: pedagogies, practices, resistance. Bloomsbury Methuen, London

Ritzer G (2004) The McDonaldization of society. Sage, London

Rogers C (1961) On becoming a person, a therapist's view of psychotherapy. Houghton-Mifflin, Boston

Simplican S (2015) Care, disability, and violence: theorizing complex dependency in Eva Kittay and Judith Butler. Hypatia 30(1):217–233

Sloan C (2018) Understanding spaces of potentiality in applied theatre. Res Drama Educ : The Journal of Applied Theatre and Performance 23(4):582–597

Stanislavski C (1990) An actor's handbook. Methuen, London

Taylor N, Wyres M, Green A, Hennessy-Priest K, Phillips C, Daymond E, Love R, Johnson R, Wright J (2021) Developing and piloting a simulated placement experience for students. Br J Nurs 30:13

Thompson J (2009) Performance affects: applied theatre and the end of effect. Palgrave Macmillan, Basingstoke

Thompson J (2023) Care aesthetics: for artful care and careful art. Routledge, London

Titchen A, Cardiff S, Biong S (2017) The knowing and being of person-Centred research practice across worldviews: an epistemological and ontological framework. In: McCormack B, Dulmen S, Eide H, Skovdahl K (eds) Person-Centred healthcare research. Wiley-Blackwell, Chichester, pp 31–51

Tizzard-Kleister K, Jennings M (2020) "Breath, belief, focus, touch": applied puppetry in simulated role play for person-centred nursing education. Appl Theatre Res 8(1):73–87

Umathum S (2015) Actors, nonetheless. In: Umathum S, Wihstutz B (eds) Disabled theatre. Diaphanes, Berlin, pp 99–112

White M (2009) Arts development in community health: a social tonic. Radcliffe, Oxford

Overcoming Vulnerability

6

Introduction

This chapter will present and discuss the findings that comprise my doctoral study's second main theme: 'overcoming vulnerability'. In the first instance, this theme highlights some of the barriers that seemed to hinder the participants in my study from moving towards performing person-centred care. These barriers appeared to be formed by deep, complex, and interwoven feelings of fear and anxiety felt by the majority of the participants in different ways. By engaging with these feelings through discussions and activities, the course put these sensations in the spotlight. This chapter will explore how, by engaging in the drama course and having these feelings highlighted rather than avoided, the group could better identify specific vulnerabilities in themselves and others. They also demonstrated a comprehension that some of these vulnerable feelings are based almost entirely on personally constructed internal fears and anxiety, rather than any external concern.

This chapter tells the thematic story of how the group developed an awareness of how to recognise, challenge, and overcome these feelings through participating in drama-based activities. The practical, interactive, and relationship-focused approach of the course served to provide a psychologically safe space in which to encounter and explore personal vulnerabilities. Moreover, the group were able to challenge their vulnerabilities in specific and 'risky' ways. This seemed to make the participants feel more confident in taking part in these, and future, activities. This growth in confidence was partnered with creative flourishing, which the course promoted and fostered. The last stages of this chapter and the story of this theme look at how the group became comfortable with the uncomfortable through engaging in dramatic activity. This includes role plays which developed in complexity and challenge over time and as the participants became more used to performing in them. As mentioned earlier, this development was aided by a strong sense of safety alongside purposeful challenges in the course.

© The Author(s), under exclusive license to Springer Nature Switzerland AG 2024

K. Tizzard-Kleister, *Applied Drama and Person-Centred Nursing*, https://doi.org/10.1007/978-3-031-77208-5_6

Providing Psychological Safety to Help Realise Vulnerabilities

Many participants reported feeling anxious when attending the first session of the course. It appeared that for some these nerves were severe, causing a sense of fear along with the conscious use of coping mechanisms, such as forced laughter.

> *I felt very nervous about coming to this today. At first I was scared and giggled a lot*
> (Gabrielle: 13–14)

Though initially tentative, the environment of the course fostered and nurtured trust leading to participants expressing things they would not have expressed otherwise. A call for creating and respecting trusting environments and relationships echoes from both literature in person-centred nursing and literature in applied, social, and participatory performance. Titchen et al. (2017), for instance, describe attempts to create PCN environments which are 'as relaxed, calm, psychologically safe and trusting as possible' (p. 36). Whilst Dewing and McCormack (2015) advocate for the increased focus on PCN approaches such as engagement to 'engender trust and so enable people to work together more effectively' (p. 2). Mirroring this, participatory performance has sought to reimagine the performer/spectator relationship in terms of trust and co-creation. For instance, exploring situations where the 'participants enter the unfamiliar using trust' whilst the performer reciprocally trusts the participant with 'the structure' of the performed encounter (O'Grady 2017: p. 1). These arguments resonate powerfully with the findings of my research study. I argue that the drama-based approach used in my study provided a trusting space for the participants, as called for by PCN researchers. Meanwhile, the course gave the group a space to work through and within the reciprocal and mutually interdependent trusting relationships that give life to engaging participatory performance practice. As a result, participants were open to sharing important aspects of themselves with the facilitators and each other, helping them to address feelings of vulnerability with the support of those around them.

The participants were tasked with performing as characters who felt a variety of emotions in SRPs. However, it appeared that in the early stages of the course, the dominant expression by the participants whilst in their roles was feelings of vulnerability. These sensations were not displaced into the character being performed but felt by the participants as actors within the scenes. These vulnerable feelings made it harder for the participants to perform as characters and engage in the role play. A particular sense of anxiety was evident when participants played the part of a nurse in SRP, which was a sense of anxiety not expressed for any other role. This anxiety seems similar to the feelings reported by the participants whilst on clinical duty. This anxiety was reported to be reduced by certain factors, such as wearing their nursing uniform like armour. However, it did not appear that the uniform or job role granted them the same protection in the SRPs as it did in real life.

> *today I play the role of a nurse.*
> *It made me feel anxious.*
> *[...]*

as the patient I felt vulnerable (Jamie: 717–719, 797)

The group expressed an understanding of the notion of vulnerability—describing the vulnerabilities they encountered and experienced through certain activities as well as a theoretical idea of it. In some reflections, such as Jamie's below, this concept was related to a nursing context, specifically the vulnerability one may feel when unwell.

<u>Vulnerable</u> - *means to feel less of who you were when you were well. Alone, isolated, unsure of what is happening or exposed* (Jamie: 407–408)

The findings of this study suggest that the creative approach of the course helped participants to engage in and address personal vulnerabilities and so increased their confidence. It is widely held that applying drama to healthcare and nursing helps to promote creativity or innovation in a field dominated by a critical paradigm (Brodzinski 2010; McCullough 2012; Dümenci and Keçeci 2014). The findings from this research study suggest that one main way the participants overcame personal vulnerability and anxiety was through engaging in creative practice. This suggests that engaging with creative practice over a longer duration may be useful beyond simply developing 'creative and critical-reflexive skills' to help in the day-to-day activity of nursing as de Oliviera et al's study of the benefit of SRP in nursing students argues (2015: p. 54).

In my drama course, creative approaches included a deeper engagement with, and sharing of, sometimes difficult personal feelings. This meant that participants had more sensitive exchanges, contributing to the cultivation of creative skills in natigating these interactions. For example, the application of actor training techniques meant that the participants felt less vulnerable during face-to-face interactions and more empowered to be creative and expressive in these exchanges. This is linked to how applying improvisation into practical work for non-arts-based staff reportedly enhances the gamut of creative responses the participant has access to in work and everyday life (Dudeck and McClure 2018). What the findings of my study point towards alongside the findings of studies like Dudeck and McClure's (2018) is the benefit of specific and rigorous approaches to creative practice as a potent amplifier of inter-disciplinary practices and personal growth. In this case, the application of actor training approaches served to amplify the participants' ability to communicate. In one major way, this was achieved by moving away from seeing communication (and person-centred nursing skills more broadly) as innate traits to seeing them as skills and features which are cultivated and developed over time. This undercut the group's reported sense of vulnerability when considering that 'being a good nurse' is intrinsically tied to what they perceived as attributes of themselves they felt were weak, and unchangeable. For example, and grossly oversimplifying, one may (perhaps rightly) think that 'being a good nurse' means being a good listener. Therefore, thinking that you are not a good listener may make you feel you are not a good nurse. As a result, considering your ability to listen as a trait that is not developable means you can never be a good nurse. This would cause understandable and deep feelings of vulnerability. What the application of actor training helped with was providing an approach to developing skills which are often seen more as innate traits and virtues. Simply, this helped the participants see how they could challenge their vulnerability of themselves as lacking, to see the potential they had to flourish.

It seemed that the experience of different forms of personal and general vulnerability in the sessions prompted a deeper awareness of how participants might feel that way, as explored by participants in insightful personal reflections. It seemed that in some cases, the participants reflected on personal feelings and vulnerabilities in a more creative and aesthetic tone than other topics. Using a creative mode of reflection promoted and facilitated the participants to express and explore these types of sensations in ways that more critically based reflections might not have. Perhaps this is due to creative methods helping to push boundaries more gently and diffusely.

> *I felt like they were seeing the real me through my eyes and I didn't like* [sic]. *I hide my true self from people and with that task I felt very unprotected and like I was standing on a cliffside in the fog.* (Hannah: 194–197)

By focusing on mutual, interactive, and dialogic learning in an emotionally trusting environment, the drama course contributed to the participant's engagement with the emotional and affective work of nursing. Moreover, it invited challenging critical discourse through the prism of creative practice. The shift to seeing the emotional work of nursing incited by the course emerged through the in-process affective dimension of the creative arts. This resonates with the aesthetics of care, which repositions the aesthetics in applied drama practice into the relationships and mutual care performed by those involved in the project. It could be argued that the course modelled an environment characterised by Thompson's notion of an aesthetics of care, where it focused on the 'aesthetics built in the sensations stimulated in the particular moment' (Thompson 2015: p. 439). Aligning with Arrighi et al. (2018) this promoted a 'situation-driven' rather than 'goal-driven' approach to educational SRP.

The participants explored these aesthetic moments and in so doing articulated learning points to apply in the future. This suggests that practically engaging in the affective and emotional aspects of nursing may significantly benefit the student nurse. This accords with how the PCNF argues that seeing care '*as an affect* emphasises the nature of the emotional involvement in caring', further suggesting person-centred care has an inherent aesthetic quality capable of moving our emotional and sensuous faculty (McCormack and McCance 2010: p. 25). The implication here is that this aspect of nursing work is directly addressed and, in many ways, enhanced through the drama course.

By centralising the affective nature of the work through an aesthetics articulated between and in relation to people, the drama course seemed to tackle the use of emotional 'numbing as a cognitive defence against intense affect that prevents emotional processing' (Leahy 2002: p. 187–8). This is described in Leahy's study on emotional processing to lead to 'greater emphasis on rationality, less control, and blaming others for emotions' (Ibid). This supports the arguments of a wide array of applied drama theorists who explore the unique and potent nature of affect in applied drama practices as both an aesthetic and pedagogic experience (Tait 2021). For instance, Brodzinski asserts that one of the most important aspects of theatre in healthcare is how 'the affective experience' creates 'a point of 'real' connection for an audience' (2010: p. 150). This may lead the audience/participant to make a change or engage with a topic more robustly. Cathy Sloan, exploring the potential of applied drama in the context of addiction recovery, concludes that in an applied drama space characterised by potentiality, '[a]ffect can then be considered as a philosophical concept of our body's capacity for acting in the world' (2018: p. 584). Returning to the exploration of vulnerability as our experience of being moved from one stable point to another in Part 1, I add to Sloan's apt statement that applied drama spaces characterised by potentiality are spaces in which we can act, and be acted upon. More precisely, in applied drama spaces, we are moved and move others through the language of 'affect', shared amongst people through sensation and presence in a live and dialogic interplay. It is this two-way process that Prentki (2023) gestures towards as a distinct feature of how drama and theatre works both intersubjectively and intra-subjectively.

This 'capacity for acting' was not gained without a struggle. The group identified a fear of failure through not wanting to say or do the wrong thing in 'risky' situations—even in a simulated environment—as a powerful barrier. At times, this fear had a paralysing effect, causing participants to stop and focus singularly on what they thought would be the correct, or even perfect, response rather than responding in the moment.

> Gabrielle: you do think on your toes, like. [over top of each other] Like when -
> Rowan: You have to think quick -
> Gabrielle: someone says a question to you, you're like right what do I need to say here – like you do think. If you don't know why, I would just say gimme two minutes- (Focus group: 1403–1408)

The course served to highlight a particular fear in the participants which could be said to be shared by the majority of early-stage nursing students—the fear of making a mistake. The participants of this course began the workshops feeling that failure was wholly negative and that the nefarious consequences of failure far outweighed the learning one might gain from this moment. Some studies highlight how drama is particularly effective at exposing nursing students' seemingly inherent fear of failure. For Dingwall et al. (2017) nursing, when compared to other similar professions, is a field that can be described to be over securitised in terms of risk-taking. They highlight this as a significant barrier for nursing students to engage with person-centred approaches.

During the early stages of the course, failure marked an endpoint—a 'full stop'—for the participants. In their initial interactions, they felt what they were offering was too dangerous a risk, and so failure was not an option. This sensation characterised their interactions, their engagement with every aspect of the course and arguably their attendance at the course itself. However, over time the content and delivery of the course made failure, however, big or small, feel less threatening and dangerous, more of a comma than a full stop. What the group seemed to develop was a deeper understanding of avoidance, and indeed how to *avoid avoidance*. Arguably, this is due to a particular strength of the drama-based pedagogy, namely that drama-based practices readily accept mistakes. In some cases, mistakes are sought out and celebrated as *better* than the original intention. Entire fields of performance practice are dedicated to this idea in what has become broadly termed the 'poetics of failure'. This is an area of performance where genuine and ephemeral moments emerge almost at random from passing through instances of designed, semi-designed, or non-designed failure in performance. Echoing Samuel Beckett, Sara Jane Bailes describes how exploring failure with both a critical and creative eye exposes aspects of '[t]he human condition; that there is nothing to express, not the means to express, and yet the compulsion to express' (2010: p. 1). The participants exemplified this in their reflections, discussions, and interactions—where even without the means to express what they wished to, their tenacity to make the effort to do so grew and grew. They discovered a new improvisational language that did not fear a mistake but used the mistake as generative creative material for the role play.

For the participants, it could be said that accepting failure opened up the vast potential of embodied encounters. As Barton and Hansen (2017) explore, failure is made to work as an aesthetic collaborator in some contemporary performance practices. Failure can thereby be seen as a moment of creative intervention which opens a 'multiplicity of possible futures afforded by failure' itself (Ibid: p. 133). Taking this into account, I argue that the drama course offered the participants a space to feel failure without the threat or risk of danger or harm, in turn improving their ability to interact with others with openness and generosity. The result of this acceptance of failure was increased confidence in making creative choices, and in particular, taking creative risks.

Cultivating Creative Confidence

Frequently, vulnerability and personal difficulties such as anxiety and nervousness were navigated using the idea of the nursing uniform as protection. This protection seemed to secure a personal and individual sense of stability as well as facilitate an ability to compartmentalise and numb your concerns and emotions for the sake of others.

> They describe to us that when they are in uniform, on the ward, they feel completely differently. They use the word armour to describe this. (Field notes: 1215–1217)

Without this armour, it seemed that taking part in risky activities, particularly activities involving personal and emotional engagement, caused discomfort for many of the participants. At first, during exercises that looked at the risk of failure in different ways, the group seemed to focus all their attention on the moment of failure. This illustrated the fear they had of making mistakes, along with the discomfort this could produce. By exploring the exercises and discussing failure as transitory the group's focus shifted to the objective at hand and the people involved rather than what could go wrong. This improved the performance of the group in the drama activities, and their role plays.

> *After a few goes around the focus intensifies and the group react to each "failure" with more vested interest. I explain that the focus is great, but we need to think of the moments of failure a little more. Instead of seeing that failure as a big deal, which we have to react to, to acknowledge it, and return to the task whilst maintaining our focus. A couple of attempts later, by using this focus, we manage it!* (Field notes: 1374–1380)

It became clear that participants were able to recognise their fears and the effect that fear may have on them. It was demonstrated by the group and eloquently reflected on individually by Jamie, that fear is often based on perception, and the effects this has subjectively can drastically overemphasise the danger behind a fear.

> *Fears - we all have different fears. It depends on your perception of something or what you know about something or what someone has told you. Sometimes we catastrophise fears because of anxiety - but they turn out to be not as bad as you thought initially* (Jamie: 410-413)

Instead of creating more anxiety and making it harder for the group to take part, it appeared that purposefully adding elements of difficulty for the group to navigate opened up these feelings for the participants to consider and work through productively. These feelings were acknowledged, normalised, and worked through, not avoided. Tasks such as focusing only on your partner's eyes for an extended duration or simulating an awkward exchange between a nurse and their patient seemed to bring up a variety of striking feelings for the group. It seemed that by encouraging the participants to focus both on completing these tasks and engaging in the powerful feelings they brought up, the participants were better able to openly discuss and eventually address these feelings and any difficulties related to the exercise, and potentially future practice.

> *in this session, I believe I took a lot more from it. One aspect that really stood out was the task at the end that you had to hold hands with your partner and look at them in the eyes. Once hearing that the eyes were the same eyes whether they were a baby or whether they were old, really struck me.* (Gabrielle: 89–93)

Drama practitioners and teachers are well used to open dialogue based on feelings with groups. The participants were often asked questions like 'How did that activity make you feel?', 'Why did you react that way?', 'How could we change this to make it feel different?', and so on. It was fairly evident that the group were not used to questions like this in their studies. Discussions like these were informed and energised by the embodied activities. It was often the activity, and the participant's bodily experiences of the activity, that sparked lively exchanges in the group. Other activities seemed to have similar effects. For example, participants were tasked to perform counter-intuitive actions and to respond to them in SRPs and in some drama-based activities such as 'the yes game', where two people interact with one asking for something outlandish and the other having to say yes to it (this is Chris Johnston's 'Yes Game', see Johnston 1998). Through actively performing various counter-intuitive actions, such as 'agreeing' to something you do not want to, participants explored difficult interactive methods. Although sometimes playful, these situations could also be serious and difficult to navigate, such as a simulated patient's condition worsening whilst a family member is focused on arguing with the attending nurses. Participants were tasked to overcome their concerns to help others. This served as a precursor to a later exploration of how these concerns should not be entirely numbed, as these concerns shape one's personhood and often help define who we feel we are and how we engage with others.

> *I also secretly task Rowan and Alice with making PJ convulse and shake uncontrollably if the scene devolves into an argument.* (Field notes: 1695–1697)

Puppetry applied to the mannequins challenged the group to keep attending to their patient whilst engaging with other competing concerns that (often rightly and understandably) demanded their attention. These included agitated family members, issues with team members, demands on time, working through restrictive bureaucratic policies which—though incredibly important—increased demand on individuals at the moment, and more. Hulkko and Laakkonen (2022) describe how through puppetry an actor locates their centre outside of themselves when performing, and so they 'exercise material sensibility' (p. 318–319). The participants discovered how difficult it is to maintain a responsive performance of sympathetic presence, though by actively relocating their centre to their patients they could better attend to their patient's needs in distracting situations. This was heightened when the patient was a mannequin who could not talk. For example, during the group's initial attempts to perform as the attending nurse in these scenarios, the participants responded to the increasing discomfort and confrontational approach of a simulated family member by flooding them with information. Meanwhile, they also began shifting their attention away from the mannequin until they were solely focused on the interaction with the 'problematic' family member. Through the role plays with mannequins animated by a puppeteer, with a multitude of loud and distracting activities as the backdrop, the participants learned how to approach these confusing and difficult situations. They learnt how to use different forms of communication and interpretations of meaning than verbal ones to continue performing sympathetic presence with the others in their interactions. This included seeing listening as an action, an active process that takes effort to do well.

Performance theorist Heddon (2017) explains that as only humans were historically considered capable of speech, speaking up was designated as an affirmation of anthropocentric political agency. The implication for Heddon, who searches for a more inclusive approach to participative performance practice, is to imbue 'mute subjects' with agency by listening deeply. 'To be a deep listener is surely to be a resonant subject sensing beyond meaning' (2017: p. 32). The participants expressed a deeper awareness of listening, as well as giving voice to others beyond the voice of verbal language through interacting with mannequins as simulated patients. In this case, we meet each person where they are, rather than assert the primacy of speech as a designator of worth and agency. For example, just because a family member has a greater capacity for speech than a patient, that certainly does not mean this family member's contributions have more worth and agency than their kin. Making shared decisions is not just a verbal act. Listening as an interactive and often non-verbal action promotes an equalised power dynamic and affirms the agency all people should have regarding their health and well-being.

Engaging with challenging situations as well as purposefully counter-intuitive actions as learning processes seemed to provide an experience of the feelings involved when doing or saying something perhaps considered taboo for the participants. The experience of contradictory and difficult interactions prompted a heightened awareness of body language, and how someone's presence communicates. The embodied experience of this 'negative' interaction demonstrated the effect of such actions on the participants, who were able to identify and express the importance of this type of communication. It also made it clear that though you may feel you are expressing what you wish to express when chiefly concerned with other things like personal anxiety or fear, these expressions are more and more unconsciously influenced by that than we realise.

> *Hannah: I think the negative body language thing that you did, like walking up to somebody, like the way Matt walked up like he was gonna hit you, but then he spoke calmly [laughter] like a mixed signal kind of thing. I think that shows you like - your body language speaks more than your verbal does to somebody.*
> *Nic: speaks a thousand words*
> *[general agreement]* (Focus Group: 396-402)

The experience of a previous interaction in a past situation, whilst helpful for a sense of personal confidence, may not necessarily offer an effective solution or approach to the one they face there and then. This is the greatest difference between the training necessary to complete technical tasks efficiently and the development of effective interpersonal skills. When learning a technical skill, the aim is to replicate and repeat the task correctly, which must be performed in the same way each time. It is a repeatable and replicable *transaction*. In contrast, the completion of an interpersonal skill relies on the opposite. Arveklev et al.'s (2015) review highlights how drama opens 'the possibility to get in the role as fictive patients and relatives and thereby explore different perspectives' (p. 17). Drawing from this suggestion, the participant's experience of the patient's role in the drama course highlighted how the nurse presents themselves and how different presentations might make the patient feel concerning how that nurse presents. It also affirmed that no encounter is the same so no single approach will fulfil the demands of every interaction. Each interaction requires active *translation* of the situation and presented selves involved (Tizzard-Kleister and Jennings 2020).

These experiences were memorable, offering participants direct, embodied, and sensed understandings of how to deal with different and difficult situations. It emerged that this memory was not entirely abstract or based on theoretical ways to deal with problems but had a basis as a memory of how you dealt with it. This meant the group linked their personal experiences in the exercises and SRP in which they overcame dilemmas to future practice. The experiences were inscribed within them (Nolan 2009). These activities that enabled this type of memory helped participants feel prepared and able to draw on the drama-based activities to help them in real situations.

> Alice: *Definitely. You feel prepared, once you had the simulation done, in the role plays and everything, and if it happens in real life –*
> Rowan: *you'd just think back –*
> Alice: *You'd just think back to like how it as dealt with in the group, you know, so through drama then we were able to apply it then to real life.* (Focus group: 1381–1385)

Participants commented on the calming nature of the course's delivery and how this led to open self-improvement through an increased reflective ability. The course felt like a safe environment for the group. The delivery of the course created a space where participants felt able to speak openly and discuss subjects perhaps usually ignored or avoided. This openness appeared to develop a level of trust amongst the group and the facilitators so that the group were able to show and engage in emotions and emotional content safely, particularly in light of the complex and difficult situations explored. Participants expressed a freedom to cry and to disclose things they might have kept to themselves, as they encountered and overcame barriers between themselves and others.

> Gabrielle: *that's something I have never told anybody.*
> Jamie: *I know I-*
> Gabrielle: *you know-*
> Jamie: *I didn't think I would ever cry on this drama course.* (Focus group: 481-484)

The group showed how taking part in the drama course facilitated them to be open and creative, particularly within their reflections. Though many of the reflections were general or related to identifying personal traits that might be of value in their future careers, some of the participant's reflections touched on deeply personal vulnerabilities. Interestingly, these features of the group's reflective practice throughout the course seemed to be significantly enhanced by using creative approaches. Though I am not certain enough to suggest why this was the case, speculatively I suggest it may be that creative approaches act as a diffuser to the intensity or immediacy of certain feelings.

Allen and Brodzinski (2009) explore perceptions of creativity and risk in the NHS. They highlight how many existing interventions and approaches involve a creative 'toolkit that explores the known [and] may not allow for creativity in terms of invention and exploration', in turn 'serving a more controlling function' than was intended or is useful (p. 314). This critique is particularly relevant concerning the findings of my study. In particular, how engaging in less controlled creative approaches which rely on 'unpredictability in the process' leads to open and generous reflections that greatly support a participant's ability to overcome feelings of anxiety and fear (Ibid). These reflections were often distinctly phrased to merge aesthetic and formal language which seemingly helped the participants to define terms which were difficult to pin down in words, such as sympathetic presence. Some of the participant's technical communication skills, such as spelling and grammar, could be said to be slightly poor.[1] However, the majority of the group wrote at least one reflection which I thought was beautiful, eloquent, and evocative. What this writing expressed in ways in which more technically competent language might not be able was the sensations behind the participant's experience.

The participants began this process tentatively, initially unsure about engaging with the process of self-reflection involved. As Allen and Brodzinski (2009) highlight there is a widely held notion amongst healthcare staff 'that self-reflection, analysis and even evaluation are seen as time-wasting' (p. 315). My research study shows that this assumption as well as a perceived fear of failure is a significant barrier to developing person-centred nurses. It also suggests that the drama course prompted the participants to be engrossed in problem-solving as a group who performed care for one another as well as to confront fears and anxieties which held the participants back. This freedom of expression was observable in the content and discussion of some exercises. Exploration and openness were encouraged, with participant interpretation a central element of the course. Even 'mistakes' were explored with equal amounts of joy and seriousness, perhaps resulting in an environment where taking a risk felt safer.

> Alice says "Annie are you okay", this makes us laugh and think of the Michael Jackson song, we all have a laugh and can't stop thinking about it! Matt suggested this could even be used as a strategy [...] I say imagine presenting this to lecturers on Friday! (Field notes: 2040–2043)

This created an open space for the participants to offer their thoughts and opinions with acceptance and dialogue. It was evident that participants understood the importance of being open and discussing their issues if needed, particularly in their future profession. The group saw great value in expressing feelings and an awareness that this leads to a lessened perception of difficult emotions, isolation, and exposing feelings. This led some to express how the session had made them feel more positive about themselves, their studies, and their future profession.

Berardi (2015) explains that in a world increasingly dominated by digital information focused on the smooth connection between compatible machines, art

---

[1] I do not mean this as a judgement. I have struggled with spelling and grammar, particularly as I am more used to writing for performance, in which I write in a "vernacular" rather than a precise way. I am, and have long been, more interested in the meaning found between language, and what is lost in language, than "correct" formal articulation. I truly believe, as evidenced by the participants, that we are more able to communicate than traditional forms of accepted communication would have us believe.

practice uniquely creates conjunctions between information by opening a 'sensitive interface between the conscious self and the infinite emission of signs' (p. 39). Berardi suggests that the increase in feelings of anxiety across the social strata is a result of our perception of the world being disrupted, as systems are set up for frictionless digital connection which stall when things do not easily and immediately connect. It is through the languages of aesthetics and sensation that complex, conjunctive, understanding bypasses the problems created by incompatible ways of being in the world. The participants showed this through the drama course as they fostered and discovered creative means in which to understand and express themselves and to understand sympathetic presence. This also helped them to articulate feelings and sensations beyond the capacity of other, more cognitive, languages to define. This suggests that apart from encouraging the sharing of difficult feelings, creative approaches may also explore the sensations and emotions behind these experiences in ways that others can understand on a variety of levels. The participants' ability to detect and perform sympathetic presence was significantly enhanced through creative approaches which in turn helped them to tap into feelings and sensations, instead of relying on 'displaying' emotional states. They were more open to the 'infinite emission of signs' expressed in non-digital communication and better able to understand more of them (Ibid). For instance, the group felt emotionally connected to their peers when we explored concepts of safe space. The presence of the participants adapted in response to the generosity of their peers who were offering their feelings, and the vulnerability which they expressed. To use the language explored in Part 1, the group expressed 'conviviality' and sympathetic presence in response to the amount at which an individual revealed their own 'debility' (Calvert 2020).

Meanwhile, the participants worked together in the course to address different issues which permeated the structure of the course, creating an environment where the participants must repeatedly offer and implement solutions in exercises and role plays. At times this process of problem-solving included the participants disclosing and exploring personal and emotional things about themselves. This required the participants to cooperate with an acknowledgement that this was not a place for judgements but for acceptance and shared responsibility. This resonates with Calvert's (2020) notion of 'performance engrossment'. This is where the performers care for a performance through caring for each other as mutually interdependent people in shared 'debility', working together through 'conviviality' towards a mutual goal. Reaching a point at which a group can be engrossed in this takes time and careful guidance.

It is clear through these findings and the findings of my research project that creating spaces of potentiality (Sloan 2018) is to create a space in which individuals can explore and practice their agency. I argue, supported by the findings of this study, that nursing students must build and foster trusting relationships which thrive on openness, conviviality, and reciprocity. I argue that the drama course in my research study provided nursing students with multiple experiences of affective encounters in a process related to Thompson's articulation of the aesthetics of care.

This could become a crucial element and template for understanding the affective nature of person-centred nursing care in practice and on a wider scale.

I felt at ease and at peace with myself. The second session was fantastic. I love doing the yoga and mindfulness meditation. I feel more positive about my nursing degree as I have been struggling. (Alice: 29–34)

Studies into how student nurses engage with the emotional work of nursing, such as Heggestad et al. (2016), describe how nursing students need to learn how to 'balance between affective and cognitive' approaches to care (p. 793). In many of the exercises in the course, particularly the SRPs, emotional distancing was actively challenged and analysed. It could be argued that emotional distancing was a factor in how the participants engaged with the types of exercises and SRPs in the drama course, with some finding certain exercises challenging, or even impossible. Consequently, this type of learning may be difficult to access and engage in for those unwilling or less able to be generous and open. Alternatively, it could offer a rich method for identifying and challenging emotional distancing. I resist any move to make this process about assigning a label or blame on a person as 'open and generous' or not, especially if this leads to the subsequent logic that they can or cannot be a person-centred nurse without this openness or generosity. I am not arguing this facet of a person as an absolute identifier of their capacity to be person-centred, but that this offers a crucial opportunity to reflect on how engaging in this process significantly enhances the potential for person-centredness. What might stifle that potential is harsh judgement and perceived pressure from peers.

Arveklev et al. (2020) highlight this issue in their drama intervention into nursing education. They define the discomfort felt by some nursing student participants when tasked with engaging in drama activity as unfulfillable 'performance requirements […] from their peers when acting in the role of a nurse' (p. 5). Though there is some suggestion of this from the findings of this study, there is also evidence to suggest potential for the opposite effect, where the group worked together to elevate each other through tackling difficult feelings head-on. As explored earlier in the chapter, the group spent less time focusing on what they perceived to lack as attributes of 'a good nurse', and more time exploring their potential. In this way, drama serves to expose, explore, and overcome a participant's anxiety about 'performance requirements'. As a result, although drama activity may alienate some participants, it may also encourage these same people, through challenging collaboration and interdependence. I suggest that anxieties that are unexplored may always serve as a barrier for an early career nurse until they are addressed. The subsequent argument is that addressing these barriers in an educational simulated environment is far safer for both patients and practitioners than coming across them in a real situation. Drama-based activity might be incredibly effective for challenging and overcoming issues arising from emotional distancing and actively addressing and fulfilling performance requirements. Engaging in the drama course seemed to help the participants feel comfortable with the uncomfortable. This was not through simply having experience of that situation that they could fall back on to find their confidence from, but through the acquisition of skills and confidence in feeling equipped to cope in challenging unexpected circumstances. The drama course as a pedagogic space can therefore serve a direct tangible purpose for person-centred nursing students to explore what a person-centred nurse is, and how to be one. Moreover, the drama course can be said to have fostered interactive, dialogic, and embodied learning towards a space of potentiality where the participants tested the limits of their capacity through the language of 'affect' (Sloan 2018). This in turn shifted their perception of themselves as inescapably lacking, to perceiving their personhood as potent and always growing to better engage in the dance and interplay of the 'infinite emission of signs' that non-digital interaction with other people inherently involves (Berardi 2015: p. 39).

Becoming Comfortable with the Uncomfortable

Participants expressed increased comfort with things they have never done before as a result of taking part in the course. The course was identified as encouraging confidence by pushing the participants beyond their comfort zones. The skills explored within the drama course seemed to illustrate and facilitate personal confidence, particularly when interacting with patients. For instance, Nic (who is someone who does not appear to lack confidence) reflected on his developed personal confidence achieved through the course as well as a nuanced understanding of how showing this confidence directly relates to patient interaction and person-centred nursing.

> Nic: I'd say the drama skills we learnt just sort of made you more confident with yourself and doing things we're not comfortable with, it helps to bring you a bit more out of your comfort zone and show more confidence for yourself, and more obviously it helps to be more confident towards the patient as well. (Focus Group: 23–27)

The results of this study resonate with the powerful findings of Cathy Salit (2018) and her study into using applied improvisation with registered oncology nurses. Shared features include 'more teamwork, collegiality, and community amongst staff', enhanced ability 'to initiate and deepen relationships' as well as 'improved communication and support skills' through 'a shared language for handling the emotional impact of'—in Salit's context—'patient's dying' (2018: p. 72). Though this drama course did not follow an applied improvisation methodology, it is clear that there are deeply resonant shared outcomes and features, arguably through the somewhat shared history and 'DNA' of the two different approaches.

Participants were able to identify breathing and relaxing as methods to lower stress and through which to show their confidence and how this might benefit interactions with others. There was a sense of surprise at how useful these exercises were. For instance, many participants described how they had never considered how they breathe, the importance of breathing, or the use of certain exercises actively involving breathing and how this may reduce stress. Gabrielle even reported using these techniques she had learnt daily.

Gabrielle: I think I'd be using it more and more - every day.
Karl: Every day?
Rowan: I never thought I'd do it.
Gabrielle: If my stress levels are high.
Karl: Since the drama, you're doing it every day?
Gabrielle: I would breathe aye, I never would even have thought to -
Rowan: I'd never have thought to breath -
Gabrielle: to take time out to do it -
Rowan: I'd never think that breathing is ever gunna calm me down -
[...]
Rowan: It didn't take the stress completely away, but it just made you think -
Gabrielle: Calms you -
Rowan: think, it's gunna be OK.
[Rowan, then Jamie laughs] (Focus group: 1141–1155)

It was identified that activities and exercises that dealt with reducing stress in the nursing profession were incredibly important and perhaps underserved. The ability for an individual to be calm, relaxed, and centred was directly linked to reducing stress, increasing confidence, and also potentially improving care outcomes and delivery. This link shows how the participants had developed an understanding that acknowledging and then managing vulnerabilities leads to overcoming them, and to better performances of care in SRPs and daily work. It also highlights the skills attained to achieve this, and a recognition of the internal and external factors influencing an individual's ability to overcome fears and vulnerabilities.

- *Minor exercises like breathing can actually be seen as MAJOR exercise as it affects our psychology as well as physiology.*
- *It is these types of exercises that help prevent stress and worry that may affect our day-2-day jobs or activities.*
- *For nurses, this is a big factor that can affect how we deliver care and so, is recognised as a very important exercise* (Nic: 985-990).

The participants also discovered that the drive to complete technical tasks often masquerades as a value system. For instance, where the more efficiently one completes a technical task the more one sees them as the most valuable part of nursing practice, in turn making performing the processes from the PCNF far more difficult. This confirms McCormack and McCance's (2010) notion that reliance on a technical task-based approach increases the 'risk of undertaking physical tasks without paying attention to person-centred processes' (p. 106). A task-based focus and mechanistic environment takes attention away from the holistic needs of people involved in person-centred nursing. Although the participants began the course feeling that their time was condensed, as they were perhaps pulled towards a mechanistic paradigm, this soon changed. The importance of providing care for all of a patient's needs was a key focus of the drama course. The participants also identified how the drama course taught them that their own needs are a key part of caring for others, remarking how taking time to pause and reflect was also important to PCN. The participants discovered that they often used the need to complete a technical task as a defence mechanism in place of engaging with others in the interactions in the drama course. This experience and the learning gained through reflection could guard against this happening 'in real life'.

Conclusion

This chapter has explored the second main theme of my doctoral study; overcoming vulnerability. The story of this theme begins with the provision of psychological safety which encourages the acceptance of specific vulnerabilities. In this place of safety, creative confidence was fostered. What occurred from here was participants feeling comfortable in unexpected and challenging circumstances, which previously would have been uncomfortable. The drama course helped the participants deal with difficult emotions and resistance to participation during simulated or dramatised interactions. The concept of numbing, or emotional distancing, was a significant topic in the course and noticeable in some of the participant's reflections. This was particularly related to the role of the nurse and how they interacted with patients. There seemed to be an initial perception that the nurse needed to disregard their problems in favour of their patient's needs in certain situations. This conformed to a process of emotional distancing which may anaesthetise the nurse from the suffering of others and themselves. This could, in turn, lead to a decreased capacity for the nurse to attune to the feelings of others.

By encouraging participants to take multiple roles and centralising the role of the patient as a person the drama course offers a way to attune to feelings involved in person-centred nursing. This also responds to the suggestions from the previously explored projects of both Arveklev et al. (2015) and McAllister et al. (2013). To summarise, the course provided the group with an experience of the perspective of other people, in this case, the most insightful example being patients. It also tackles the obstacle of a task-focused mentality which McCormack and McCance (2010) argue against. The drama course seemed to take away a significant amount of 'armouring' and/or numbing that the group felt necessary to do. As a result, the participants identified the need to balance the completion of technical nursing tasks with actively engaging with others as the key to performing person-centred care. Being better able to attend to others as a result of engaging in the course is the focus of the next chapter, which explores the third main theme; 'attending to others'.

References

Allen V, Brodzinski E (2009) Deconstructing the toolkit: creativity and risk in the NHS workforce. Health Care Anal 17:309–317

Arrighi G, Irvine C, Joyce B, Kristi Haracz K (2018) Reimagining 'role' and 'character': an approach to acting training for role-play simulation in the tertiary education setting. Appl Theatre Res 6(2):89–106

Arveklev SH, Wigert H, Berg L, Burton B, Lepp M (2015) The use and application of drama in nursing education—an integrative review of the literature. Nurse Educ Today 35(7):E12–E17

Arveklev S, Wigert H, Berg L, Lepp M (2020) Specialist nursing students' experiences of learning through drama in paediatric care. Nurse Educ Pract 43:1–6

Bailes SJ (2010) Performance theatre and the poetics of failure. Routledge, London

Barton B, Hansen P (2017) Risking intimacy: strategies of vulnerability in Vertical City's *All Good Things* and *Trace*. In: O'Grady A (ed) Risk, participation, and performance practice: critical vulnerabilities in a precarious world. Palgrave Macmillan, London, pp 131–152

Berardi F (2015) And: phenomenology of the end, Semiotext(e): South Pasadena

Brodzinski E (2010) Theatre in health and care. Palgrave, Basingstoke

Calvert D (2020) Convivial theatre: care and debility in collaborations between non-disabled and learning disabled theatre makers. In: Stuart Fisher A, Thompson J (eds) Performing care: new perspectives on socially engaged performance. Manchester University Press, Manchester, pp 85–102

de Oliveira SN, Prado MLD, Kempfer SS, Martini JG, Caravaca-Morera JA, Bernardi MC (2015) Experiential learning in nursing consultation education via clinical simulation with actors: action research. Nurse Educ Today 35(2):50–54

Dewing J, McCormack B (2015) Engagement: a critique of the concept and its application to person-centred care. Int Pract Dev J. [Online] Available from: https://www.fons.org/Resources/Documents/Journal/Vol5Suppl/IPDJ_05(suppl)_06.pdf. Accessed 13 Mar 2018

Dingwall L, Fenton J, Kelly TB, Lee J (2017) Sliding doors: did drama-based inter-professional education improve the tensions round person-centred nursing and social care delivery for people with dementia: a mixed method exploratory study. Nurse Educ Today 51:1–7

Dudeck T, McClure C (2018) Applied improvisation. Methuen Drama, London

Dümenci SB, Keçeci A (2014) Creative drama: can it be used in nursing education. Int J Hum Sci 11(2):1320–1326

Heddon D (2017) The cultivation of entangled listening: an ensemble of more-than-human participants. In: Harpin A, Nicholson H (eds) Performance and participation: practices, audiences, politics. Red Globe, London, pp 19–40

Heggestad AKT, Nortvedt P, Christiansen B, Konow-Lund A (2016) Undergraduate nursing students' ability to empathize: a qualitative study. Nurs Ethics 25(6):786–795

Hulkko P, Laakkonen R (2022) Actor education, object animation and care. Theatre, Dance Perform Train 13(2):309–323

Johnston C (1998) House of games: making theatre from everyday life. Nick Hern, London

Leahy R (2002) A model of emotional schemas. Cogn Behav Pract 9:177–190

McAllister M, Reid-Searl K, Davis S (2013) Who is that masked educator? Deconstructing the teaching and learning processes of an innovative humanistic simulation technique. Nurse Educ Today 33(12):1453–1458

McCormack B, McCance T (2010) Person-centred nursing: theory and practice. Wiley-Blackwell, Chichester

McCullough M (2012) The art of medicine: bringing drama into medical education. Lancet 379:512–513

Nolan C (2009) Agency and embodiment: performing gestures/producing cultures. Harvard University Press, Harvard

O'Grady A (2017) Introduction: risky aesthetics, critical vulnerabilities, and edgeplay: tactical performances of the unknown. In: O'Grady A (ed) Risk, participation and performance practice: critical vulnerabilities in a precarious world. Palgrave Macmillan, London, pp 1–29

Prentki T (2023) A short essay on empathy, drama, and a new curriculum. Res Drama Educ 28(3):387–391

Salit C (2018) Oncology nurses creating a culture of resiliency with improvisation. In: Dudeck T, McClure C (eds) Applied improvisation: leading, collaborating and creating beyond the theatre. Methuen drama, London, pp 55–78

Sloan C (2018) Understanding spaces of potentiality in applied theatre. Res Drama Educ: The Journal of Applied Theatre and Performance 23(4):582–597

Tait P (2021) Theory for theatre studies: emotion. Methuen drama, London

Thompson J (2015) Towards an aesthetics of care. Res Drama Educ: The Journal of Applied Theatre and Performance 20(4):430–441

Titchen A, Cardiff S, Biong S (2017) The knowing and being of person-centred research practice across worldviews: an epistemological and ontological framework. In: McCormack B, Dulmen S, Eide H, Skovdahl K (eds) Person-centred healthcare research. Wiley-Blackwell, Chichester, pp 31–51

Tizzard-Kleister K, Jennings M (2020) "Breath, belief, focus, touch": applied puppetry in simulated role play for person-Centred nursing education. Appl Theatre Res 8(1):73–87

Attending to Others

7

Introduction

This chapter focuses on the third theme from my doctoral study, 'attending to others'. This third main theme shows how whilst the participants overcame their vulnerabilities (explored in the previous chapter), they developed different and increasingly effective ways to pay attention and relate to others. This chapter illustrates how the participants developed abilities to attend to others, and an appreciation of the effect of doing so for person-centred nursing. This included taking the perspective of the other into account by recognising and relating to their emotions, feelings, and concerns as distinct aspects of their personhood. This occurred both cognitively and through embodiment, as participants considered and experienced these features through role plays and activities. After this, the group considered how best to help others and how best to attend to them in a way that respected their desires and needs.

For the participants, this was seen as the initial building block for creating engaging emotional relationships, and they found a deeper consideration for interacting with the people involved at the heart of the scenario. These considerations helped participants see how instead of focusing on finding a singular technically correct approach, keeping the person at the centre of their concerns during a role play made their interactions far more effective. Engaging in the course appeared to promote a recognition of the importance of emotions and non-verbal communication in person-centred nursing. The course enhanced the acquisition and development of these person-centred communication skills. In a cyclical process, these skills helped the participants to relate to others in the first place, showing how these skills are complementary to the processes of attending to others and important for person-centred nursing. In many ways, this chapter reflects on how the participants learnt how to recognise, build, and maintain supportive and therapeutic relationships with others, primarily through paying closer attention to important aspects of others.

© The Author(s), under exclusive license to Springer Nature Switzerland AG 2024
K. Tizzard-Kleister, *Applied Drama and Person-Centred Nursing*, https://doi.org/10.1007/978-3-031-77208-5_7

Relating to the Distinct Personhood of Others

The participants demonstrated an understanding that competence includes multiple factors and levels, including an ability to engage and interact with others. They identified this as a key contributor to becoming a person-centred nurse. As the participants discovered, approaches to communication can be deeply affected by the perception that a sequential and technically focused task-based approach to work is required to be competent. As Monden et al. (2016) highlight in their study into how physicians deliver bad news to patients, 'medical education has placed more value on technical proficiency than communication skills' (p. 101). This tendency permeates nursing and healthcare education. As the findings of this study suggest, this technical focus from medical education increasingly influences and affects how early-year nursing students consider and approach nursing in simulation, and potentially in practice as well.

This resonates with Berardi's (2015) notion of phenomenology based on his distinction between connection (a digital and coded linkage) and conjunction (an emergent, non-coded, and more spontaneous form of linkage). He suggests that as language relies on coding meaning, it can be easily broken down and disjointed when the codes do not align as is often the case in messy real-life interactions. This in turn may lead to deep feelings of disconnection and isolation when more and more interaction is digitally coded. This is particularly meaningful in particular given circumstances, such as the perspective of a non-verbal patient amongst 'the machinery' of a healthcare environment. Berardi advocates for a focus on sensibility to counter this, which 'can be defined as the faculty that enables the organism to process signs and semiotic simulations that cannot be verbalised or verbally coded' (2015: p. 35). For instance, sensibility is the 'faculty' through which a nurse might look at a patient and communicate reassurance through their eyes, perhaps whilst a colleague explains a technical procedure.

Eventually, the participants were better able to maintain their focus on their simulated patient, whether this patient was performed by a mannequin or one of their peers. Rather than being focused on what they should say or do as an abstract thought in a certain situation, the participants began to performatively interact with others through sympathetic presence as a first principle. The participants who performed as family members were able to give feedback on their peers' performances, highlighting points that made them feel better or worse and giving advice to improve their peer's performance. The puppeteer had a similar ability but from the perspective of the often-neglected non-verbal patient (Tizzard-Kleister and Jennings 2020). By simulating this encounter, feeding back, and re-running it, the participants began to use different strategies. These included using 'actions', such as to calm or to observe, rather than just trying to convey as much information as possible. The depth of feeling in these encounters was visibly enhanced, whilst the ethical engagement of the participants was observably deepened.

Participants reflected on how it feels to be observed. Through this reflection, there was a demonstration of an awareness that others may feel intimidated or wary when being observed. Due to the essential need for nurses to be able to observe their patients, the group highlighted a need to be able to relate to others and their feelings to observe them sensitively and effectively.

> _Observation is similar to being aware of others. It's very important to be able to observe our patients without intimidating [-ve] them._ (Jamie: 294–295)

Observing behaviour gives us information about a person, not least how they choose to express themselves. Kontos et al. (2010) argue that drama applied to PCN in the field of dementia care 'has enormous potential to facilitate a shift from viewing behaviour as a problem to be controlled, to understanding the breadth of meaning underpinning self-expression in dementia' (p. 166). They argue that this is critical for understanding that people living with dementia are 'embodied beings deserving of dignity and worth' (Ibid). In the drama course participants developed an understanding of—and ability to use—a variety of interpersonal techniques, which included ways to better observe and interpret 'the breadth of meaning underpinning self-expression' (Ibid) in all forms of interactions with a variety of different people. This gives another observable example of sympathetic presence as a performative interaction between people, which relies on the interactive embodiment of one's presence with another person.

This ability to interact with others on a person-centred level requires 'showing sympathetic presence' for Lieshout & Cardiff (2015: p. 3). This study suggests a move from showing to performing. The shift in terminology from showing to performing signals the understanding shown by the participants that sympathetic presence requires not just one person to show it through a virtuosic act. Instead, the 'spectator'—for want of a better term—co-constructs the presence. As such, a sympathetic presence is relational, dialogic, and responsive. For instance, a nurse entering a patient's room in a hurry may have a closed presence, giving off information articulating that they do not want to be disturbed. This may make a patient hesitant to express themselves, and not wanting to agitate the nurse. They might respond with an equally closed presence. This type of closed presence is indeed a valid tactic used by some nurses as a type of triage. For instance, when a nurse knows a patient elsewhere is in a more serious condition than the one looking for their attention, they close their presence to one patient to try and make more time for others who might not have time to spare. However, the drama course illustrated that there are more tactics that one might use to achieve a similar effect, without entirely 'ignoring' or 'closing off from' a patient. It also highlighted how we can slip into communicating things unintentionally and unconsciously through our body language, our feelings, our expressions, and more. Through drama-based techniques, interactive and ephemeral moments like this can be understood, explored, and improved upon. The drama approaches often provided a framework, guide, or concrete concept to ensure the participants were communicating clearly and consciously. The point at which the participants worked together openly to create and sustain the shared feeling of sympathetic presence demonstrates this. When performing sympathetic presence, one expresses their presence through their attention and focus towards another person and the openness of the expressions which they perform, even if this expression is aimed to get away from this patient to see to another as quickly as possible.

The importance of building relationships and positive environments was highlighted in many parts of the drama sessions. The participants used teamwork to achieve mutual objectives throughout. This includes multiple instances where they created a communal sense of sympathetic presence. As Tait (2021) suggests, this is beyond an emotion, or an 'affect', but can also be called a 'mood' created by a performance and understood communally. Participants were able to express how both enhanced moods and relationships could lead to more effective person-centred nursing outcomes, not least through conscious communication to achieve an objective. Conversely, the group realised these relationships are easier to develop in a caring environment.

1. the healthcare environment is so important for the patient and the nurse. Building up a relationship using communication to get your objective. (Alice: 438–440)

In this research study, the participants seemed to concurrently reflect on the perspectives of others whilst experiencing something resonant with that original experience themselves. This is through engaging in what Boal (1998) calls 'metaxis,' where one engages in reality and an image of reality simultaneously. Metaxis is identified as an important feature by many studies analysing the intervention of drama in nursing, including those of McAllister et al. (2013), Arveklev et al. (2015), and Arrighi et al. (2018). For Arveklev et al. (2015) metaxis is crucial to move simulation training beyond the acquisition of skills. Arveklev et al. (2015) highlight the importance of the use of 'dramatic context […] in order to illuminate some truth about the world' through simulated role-play, allowing those involved to engage 'in both the real and fictional contexts at the same time' (p. 13). The findings of this study support this position, where the participants felt as though they were learning skills through a simulated experience which directly applied to a future real-world situation. Importantly, this included building relationships and interacting with others in a very real and present sense, albeit in a simulated situation.

Furthermore, the findings suggest that this experience promoted a sympathetic response, as the participants thought through the perspectives of others. In doing so they more closely attuned themselves to these experiences and feelings. They began to recognise that others feel and need very different things than you think they do. Participants were keenly aware of the difference between their needs and the needs of others, particularly how focusing on their own needs might make attending to the needs of others more difficult. Crucial to this is how engaging in drama activity provides opportunities to feel things, more precisely to engage aesthetically in situational contexts and specific given circumstances in a live and embodied manner. It was clear that this focus on sensation highlighted how presence could be defined and felt, and ultimately to be used to affect how one interacts with others.

Some exercises seemed to incite responses in which participants reportedly felt the experiences of others. In some cases, participants related to others through their actions. As a result, they built closer relationships with these others through an enhanced ability to pay attention to them, being better able to identify aspects of these others like individual moods, desires, and unique needs. The usefulness of improvisation was expressed, suggesting an awareness that formulaic approaches are less appropriate or effective at achieving objectives.

> Gabrielle: *Even that one, I was the patient and I was shouting and you [To Alice] were having a fight or something? It does show you if somebody's not [...] how somebody would feel. Like, then when you came in and I challenged you on it?*
>
> *[...]*
>
> Gabrielle: *And then, a lot of people don't wanna get washed in the morning.*
>
> Rowan: *Aye.*
>
> Gabrielle: *Whereas, then, you've just kinda like, what can have to say to make them wash.*
>
> *[general agreement]*
>
> Gabrielle: *But, like in a nice way like.*
>
> Jamie: *Yeah, you have to like, improvise.*
>
> Gabrielle: *Aye, uhuh, that's what it is* (Focus group: 583–586, 1410–1418)

The drama course offered opportunities to embody sensations which were not the participant's own (or more precisely, not their habitual sensations), which led to a deeper understanding of the experiences and perspectives of others and how sympathetic presence can be performed to interpret these sensations. For instance, whilst performing as a puppeteer during a role-play or exercise some participants reported a heightened and embodied awareness of the perspective of their imagined patient through their physical and emotional connection to the object, the 'puppet'. This was also present in other drama-based exercises such as 'slow walks'. Through a mix of physical action and imaginative consideration for others, the participants seemed to transpose the experiences of others into the physical exercises they took part in during the course. This meant that the participants felt as though they were experiencing something similar to what others might experience—such as those less able to walk. This sounds closer to empathy than sympathetic presence.

It should be clear through this book so far that sympathetic presence is different from empathy, and that empathy has pitfalls that are often ignored or misunderstood. This study argues for the use of sympathetic presence in person-centred nursing. In doing this, I do not intend to reject empathy outright. Empathy can certainly be useful, though the findings of this study highlight how empathy might be better as a first step, a process of taking in the perspective of another. The next step, I argue, is crucial and must involve the principles of a well-performed sympathetic presence to enable person-centred nurses to be emotionally engaged, but protected from the insistence that they 'truly' understand and feel what others are going through to be competent. Reeves et al. (2021) consider empathy alongside imagination, borrowing from Rogers and others to suggest how empathy involves an imaginative perspective taken from one person to another. This conception of empathy includes the implication that one cannot understand and feel the experience and feelings of another, but that we can imagine them. I argue, following Hojat (2009), that this definition moves away from empathy and towards sympathy. Reeves et al.'s (2021) notion of empathy is useful as a first step. My study has shown how the participants attended to others with increased imagination and acuity, thanks to the activities undertaken. This was their first step into the lifeworlds of others.

As the related studies of Lepp (2002), Ekebergh et al. (2004) and Arveklev et al. (2018) highlight, drama can help students to consider their own and others' 'lifeworlds'. More specifically, these studies broadly explore how the lifeworld of one person might tacitly interact with the lifeworld of another, in spaces where 'all knowledge is embodied knowing' shared in a given experience (Ekebergh et al. 2004: p. 623). It could be argued that by engaging in action-oriented drama activity, the participants of this research study were encouraged to simulate the experience of others enhancing their 'embodied knowing'. In turn, the participants applied this new embodied knowledge to a rerun of the same situation, as well as the next exercises, displaying ownership of this knowledge of others, and an enhanced agency through their bodily (inter)action within the world (Nolan 2009).

By thinking of and attempting to experience the situations of other people, the participants reported sympathising with the experiences of others. For example, Gabrielle took part in an activity where the group were tasked with walking as slowly as possible. This activity led Gabrielle to equate her experience with that of her grandmother, who can only walk slowly. As a result, she sympathised with her Grandmother's experience. It appeared that participants could relate to others in this way through sensations, feelings, cognition and physicality.

Gabrielle has a moment during the slow walks, which she reports at the end during the discussions of the exercise, where she was thinking and feeling through the experiences of her grandmother who lives with dementia. (Field notes: 283–286)

I argue that an adaptable and responsive presence which can engage in dialogue with others is the basis for every caring exchange characterised by sympathy. Skovdahl and Dewing (2017) look at how we might conduct person-centred research that encourages flourishing. They raise that it is not through 'theories and views' that we relate to and 'shape' the lifeworlds of those we care for, 'but by our very presence towards him or her' (p. 88). This is where, for instance, the attending nurse responds to the presence of their patient with a practiced and performed presence, opening up a reciprocal dialogue between them. When considering Skovdahl & Dewing's assertion, this dialogue needs to be open, responsive, and sympathetic from the start to facilitate positive and effective person-centred nursing. I argue this is useful in research as Skovdahl & Dewing suggest, but also vital in every person-centred interaction. The example of Gabrielle's slow walks experience above shows the potential that embodying the experience of others has as a learning experience to better achieve and maintain a more sympathetic presence towards others. It is evident that the participants felt, experienced, and performed sympathetic presence. However, it remains that identifying specific features which explain the experience of sympathetic presence is more difficult. What is clear is that participating in drama-based activities, imagining the experience and embodiment of others, and partaking in discussions exploring person-centred ideas, contributed to an increased receptiveness to emotional relationships through engaging interactions.

Building Engaging Emotional Relationships

It seemed common for the participants to associate sympathetic presence with emotion and an ability to recognise and relate to emotions. The course provided spaces in which participants could explore their relationship with emotions by experiencing and reacting to the—sometimes intense—emotions of others. There was an appreciation of these experiences as ways to prepare for unknowable, deeply emotional future experiences, for instance, the death of a patient. Though it was rightly recognised that nothing can truly prepare you for the intensity of situations such as these, the group were aware that their experiences in the drama course (in particular, the role plays featuring emotive and challenging situations) act as stepping stones towards that experience. The application of drama in these circumstances prompted the group to confront and recognise their responses to both their own and other's emotions and to directly engage with what this feels like in a live encounter. This is not simply imagining what you might feel or watching a video or live demonstration and responding to that. It is a live, interactive, embodied, and experienced situation. In this way, the emotions are 'real' or 'authentic'. Alongside this 'real' experience is the knowledge that these situations are designed with a purpose in mind, often to prepare for the reality of person-centred nursing practice. Interestingly, the context for this live encounter did not always have to be nursing-related to feel useful in future nursing situations for the participants.

> Jamie: at the time I was feeling sad, you know. I suppose you made me think about if I was on the ward and there was an emotional situation, how would I cope with it?
> Rowan: I thought the exact same, I thought if I can't deal with my emotions here in this room listening to other people's stories how the hell am I gonna tackle -
> Jamie: I know -
> Rowan: someone dying on a ward.
> Gabrielle: you have to. (Focus Group: 488–495)

The emotions of others were identified as affective, with many participants commenting on their feelings changing in response to the feelings expressed by others in the course. Some experienced profound emotions when considering and recognising the feelings of others. The drama course was identified as beneficial to future nursing practice in terms of working with emotions. This included the emotions of others as well as one's emotional response to your work. As McCormack and McCance (2010) identify, and confirmed in the participants' experiences, a task-focused approach is a significant obstacle for a nurse to meet the prerequisites for person-centredness. For the PCNF, one prerequisite for a person-centred nurse is being 'professionally competent'. This competence is not only in technical tasks. Rather, the person-centred nurse should also have 'competence in a number of different levels that enables engagement with patients/clients and their families' (Ibid: p. 46). The findings of this course strongly suggest a key element of professional competence for the PCN is the ability to work with and through the emotions of others and their own. It is telling that working with emotions is not a more explicit feature of the NMC standards (NMC 2018), with scant mention of the emotional nature of nursing work in the standards of practice. Emotions and the specific and challenging part they play in nursing work is often assumed or ignored. PCN can be said to be an attempt to bring the human as a person into the centre of healthcare, including the emotions of both patient and practitioner.

It is clear that the activities in the drama course gave us a potential space (Sloan 2018) within which to explore emotions and our relationships with them. Working through a notion of creative engagement as openness and generosity, aligning with the notion of a congenial space (White 2009), the participants were not obliged to act on this potential. Moreover, these activities provided experiences that the group had not encountered or imagined, they were purposeful dilemmas (Preston 2016). This space provided them with an opportunity to explore how it feels to care for others through caring for each other whilst confronted with these situations. For instance, Rowan recounted how she felt during an exercise, commenting on how the emotions of her fellow participants affected her and how she linked this sensation to how she might deal with her future patient's feelings. This suggests that by interacting with another person and paying attention to their feelings during this interaction, the participants experienced how they may be affected by these interactions in an imagined future nursing context. A non-prescriptive creative approach left the door open to the participants, but the intent was never to push them through it. More so, the drama space interweaving the congenial, dilemmatic, and potential through creativity and risk-taking characterised by generosity and reciprocity facilitated the group to explore practical ways in which to navigate complex and challenging topics. To—borrowing Haraway's term—'stay with the trouble' (2016).

> Rowan: Like, I know whenever we done that, remember, it was in here, that safe place, like, we cared for everyone in the room the same way you would care for a patient, like you felt their pain, ended up crying and stuff, treating them the same if they're a patient. So like, that drama definitely got me thinking of how I'd act if someone started crying in front me that day. Cause you don't really think about how you're gunna cope until it happens, and then, whereas that kinda prepared you in a way you know. (Focus group: 1372–1379)

Skills that the drama course attempted to cultivate such as pausing, contemplating, and paying attention to one's surroundings were initially seen by the group as less important than learning through specifically designed role plays. However, after addressing the course design as an incremental build-up in a candid dialogue with the participants these skills became more and more important. This is also reflective of the group's growing engagement with the course. It could be argued that an appreciation of interpersonal skills is an ethical priority. The realisation of the cohort of the importance of these skills could be referred to as an ethical awakening, for example, when Gabrielle chose to recognise the personhood of her nonverbal, non-mobile patient through incredibly minimal cues. This was achieved by actively acknowledging this patient's personhood through Gabrielle forming a dialogue with his embodied presence. He did not have to perform a gesture to 'prove' his personhood, and so his 'worth' for person-centred care. Neither did Gabrielle give him personhood, she respected the person who was present in any way she could. Though dependent on the care of others, Gabrielle ensured her patient was treated with dignity and respect in her interactions with him, and even acknowledged his potential agency. Her actions and presence *responded* to him as much as possible. This is an example of stated behaviour change through a new moral and ethical belief system, incited by greater awareness and development of interpersonal skills. As Simplican suggests concerning interpreting the needs of others who are dependent on you, Gabrielle deciphered 'unspoken interests, desires, and projects' from her patient's perspective (2015: p. 220). As a result of the drama course, Gabrielle felt more able to *act* and to *react,* even with a person who does not give clear responses if any—effectively putting person-centred care into action.

This in turn highlights a clear difficulty also raised by Doolen et al.'s (2016) work reviewing clinical simulation practices for nursing education, namely how it is difficult to 'establish a cause-and-effect relationship' between the 'simulated learning' and actual learning outcomes and actualisation in practice (p. 301). Though it was not the purpose of the drama course to measure any causal effect on how the participants practiced nursing in a clinical setting after taking part in the drama course, this phenomenon indicates the potential to research this further in future projects. This study focused on the participant's perceptions of their understanding of PCN and their ability to embody sympathetic presence after receiving drama-based education. In this instance, I argue that a direct cause–effect relationship has taken place. For example, Gabrielle reported that her shift in caring action whilst on clinical placement was a direct response to the drama course as well as the participant's observably enhanced interactions within the course. Over the years of this study and the years after, I have observed, heard about, and researched many incredible instances of behaviour change due to the application of drama practice to a nurse's work. Finding a way to capture the impact of this phenomenon is a major area of interest for me as a researcher, and could light a path towards understanding the complex and widespread outcomes of engaging in drama for nursing students.

Participants displayed an awareness of the mutual vulnerability of patients and nurses, and how an acceptance of vulnerability can reduce anxiety and increase capacity for action. Some recognised the need for kindness in encounters with patients, showing a deeper understanding of the need to engage with others on an affective level. There was a clear engagement with the emotional perspectives of others, and the potential difficulties they may be facing, such as being unintentionally intimidated by staff, as well as ways to steer clear of perpetuating these difficulties for patients.

> *We all feel vulnerable–be empathetic, kind, and patient. Do not intimidate in an already intimidating situation.* (Jamie: 394–395)

The participants also realised the criticality for the person-centred nurse to not base their recognition of difference solely on stereotypes, traditions, or assumptions based on their feelings. This challenged their thinking about, and approach to, interactions as a transactional encounter with others. A transactional interaction serves only to achieve a task such as garnering more patient information and has no further meaning to the process of care. Instead, participants of the drama course could see how interactions predicated on person-centredness should be more closely aligned with a translational approach. Through this translational approach, the participants saw the patient not as an object through which tasks are completed, but as an equal person in an equal exchange, aligning with the notion of metaphorical translation (Tizzard-Kleister and Jennings 2020). Moreover, the healthcare tasks completed with them are not simply a means to an end but are moments of complex and interwoven caring interaction.

A specific difficulty the group felt they needed to navigate was the technical task-based focus of their work, and the resulting difficulty to pay attention to the specific needs of their patients. This technical task-first mindset included a disproportionate level of attention afforded to ensuring the correct use of specific terminology. This was a significant factor blocking or distracting individuals from engaging and interacting effectively with others in an SRP. This contributed to stilted interactions based on achieving technically focused tasks that did not relate to the patient's perspective or needs. The patient then becomes an afterthought in the process of care, which the participants reported experiencing in both SRP and clinical placement.

Alice is sympathetic as the nurse, but perhaps remains in the headspace of worrying about nursing terminology (Field notes: 2083–2085)

Gabrielle: thinking what needs done next, not thinking about -
    Jamie: Yeah, I was out on district so it was like that, thinking what to do next, instead of just – yeah.
    Rowan: Taking a moment to think about the patient afterwards like, as well.
    Jamie: Yeah. (Focus Group: 1345–1350)

As Arveklev et al. (2015) state in their review of how drama is used in nursing education, drama is well suited to exploring these ideas with nursing students to avoid the 'risk that nursing is performed as tasks or actions with no deeper meaning' (p. 12). For instance, the participants reflected on a revelation they had as a result of taking part in the drama course. This revelation revolved around understanding how as a person-centred nurse the past experiences one has are not as important as understanding or engaging with the experience of the recipient of care in that moment. Put in other terms, it was clear that they developed an awareness that just because they had nursed a patient previously with the same medical condition and a similar profile and background, does not mean that they could follow the same path with another person—saying the same things, treating them in the same approach and so on. Instead, knowledge and experience come to bear in the moment with that person, as a guide certainly, but not as a 'script'. What their experiences with drama seemed to teach them was to find the deeper meaning in each moment of performing nursing care with another person, using their nursing experience *as a person,* not just their nursing experience as a technician.

The group were able to identify how technical task-centred approaches often undermine the depth of meaning found in PCN care and the depth of interactions we have. The group highlighted how they were able to maintain attention on a patient whilst concurrently completing tasks. When participants attempted to put these ideas into practice in the SRPs they displayed a clear commitment to their patient's feelings and needs through their interactions with them. The participants used the role plays as a place in which to develop and explore these interactions, notably changing their communication approaches to achieve this. They demonstrated how communication is a skill one can learn, for example, through receiving pointed feedback on how well they comforted a patient in action in an SRP. Participants notably changed their communication to achieve this. As a result, the participants began to focus more attention on the emotional experience of their interactions. These emotional interactions were explored as a technique that could be applied to other, more abstract, situations, for example, where similar role play exercises were explored with objects and puppets.

> Rowan: Even though it's a puppet, but you're still acting like
> Karl: Yeah.
> Rowan: You cared for the puppet like [nervous laugh, then long pause]
> [...]
> Rowan: For Hannah to be taken back by that, she was so taken back, and that's probably how a doctor would feel. They would probably be like - what did I say to this woman, or her daughter?
> Gabrielle: Doctors and nurses both, anybody. (Focus group: 736–740, 1289–1292)

The group engaged in tasks that explored how the actions we perform in an inter-action convey certain information. Specifically, they realised how the way one says something affects how it is understood and received by others. As Reeves and Neilson (2018) highlight, how you say something is often more important than what you say, particularly in emotionally charged situations such as palliative and end-of-life care. The drama course provided opportunities for the participants to become more aware of, and able to develop, the contextual use of language through actions. The group saw this as hugely important, as poor interactions can cause anxiety and confusion for those they are caring for. The participants directly reported feeling this for themselves as they took part in simulations in the drama course.

The learning in the drama course seemed to not only serve the participants' ability to perform interactions with more contextual subtlety, but they also reported an enhanced sensitivity to observing and identifying different aspects of communication they may not have noticed. Participants seemed better able to provide useful feedback on their peers' performances. Throughout the drama course, this shifted from general comments on how a particular person communicated with others to noticing and suggesting more complex and specific ways the people involved in that interaction might want to interact. This signalled a clear development of person-centred communication skills.

Developing Person-Centred Communication Skills

For the PCNF 'person-centred communication is more than the sum of its parts' and 'developed interpersonal skills' is a prerequisite for a person-centred nurse. Perhaps most importantly, 'each interaction is dependent on the people involved' (McCormack and McCance 2010: p. 47). The participants in the drama course were better able to notice a wider range of meaning through self-expression in others and themselves through engaging with communication techniques which formed 'more than the sum of their parts' (Ibid). It appears the participant's experiences in the course prompted reflection and re-evaluation of the value and use of communication within nursing. This extended to the realisation that skilled use of communication is potentially lifesaving. This was coupled with an ability to see communication as simply what one says and hears in response to a more complex, multi-layered inter-action and dialogue between persons. Being open and having good communication between colleagues was also identified as one way of reducing personal stress.

> *Communication is fundamental in nursing - patient's lives literally depend on it. It is also good to communicate with colleagues - to offload after a stressful day.* (Jamie: 401–403)

Participants soon discovered that their early approaches in role plays and interac-tions drew from a smaller pool of strategies, and the potential approach to interac-tions—emotionally charged interactions in particular—was far wider than they had considered. This included the ability to adapt how they presented themselves to others, along with having a more conscious and robust understanding of the conse-quences of this presentation in terms of the effect this had on how others felt. For example, the group might not have considered using the action 'to threaten' along-side 'to calm' to help a patient understand the severity of their condition and to help them achieve their objective of calming a patient. This is analogous to Berardi's 'language of sensibility' (2015), where we open our communicative potential beyond the mechanical and towards the metaphorical. In the messy context of human interaction, intent is often misinterpreted, and cause might not lead to effect.

Features of traditional communication were explored in the sessions, with the group identifying how some patient-practitioner communication was handled poorly. One example discussed was the use of overly medical language, which might be inaccessible to many patients and can cause negative effects such as confu-sion and distancing. The participants described an awareness of the patient's needs as a person and how to adapt this medical language into clear and effective com-munication which that particular person could understand. Beyond this, the subtext of a message was highlighted in interactions. On the surface, at the level of text, there is information to convey, and ways to make it more or less understandable. At the level of subtext, however, we begin to ask questions like; how did that make the other person feel? What am I actually *doing* to them? What am I feeling about this? and so on. This led the group to consider intent, and whether what they intend to communicate is achieved, or if it is lost in the complex and often overwhelming interplay that is interpersonal communication. This prompted discussion and follow-up exercises aimed at how to be more aware of this, and how to improve and manage these ways of conveying information. This reportedly helped the participants to ensure that they were clearly and effectively communicating in the ways they wished to, with an awareness of what other people need when you speak to them.

> *Gabrielle: Because if someone spoke that medically - doctors do speak a lot, and they don't break it down for anybody.*
> *Jamie; no.*
> *Gabrielle: So it's all about - I suppose-*
> *[talking over each other]*
> *Rowan: I think that gives people more anxiety.*
> *Gabrielle: it's about good communication too and, being aware of who you're speaking to.* (Focus group: 1320–1327)

Particular attention was given to non-verbal communication. Exercises and activities in the course directly addressed the difference between the words we say, and the meaning intended behind them. Participants applied this practically, displaying increased sensitivity to the effects our bodies, our breath, and semiconscious reactions may have in communicating with others. Particularly in ways in which we may not wish to. Participants picked up on the effect that intention has on verbal communication, highlighting how meaning shifts in line with body language. Elements such as eye contact, tone, folding arms, proximity, and more were pinpointed as factors affecting non-verbal communication. The communicative potential of non-verbal forms of interaction was described as just as important, if not more important, than words.

> *Non-verbal communication*
> • *when using only two phrases today, one per person, (how are you and I'm fine) being able to use these phrases in a variety of different ways, yet mean something completely different.*
> • *Use of eye contact and a friendly, welcoming tone, "how are you?" Can be completely different/mis-interpreted to looking away with arms folded!*
> • *Our body language is just as important as words!* (Nic: 240–247)

This displayed an enhanced awareness of what Goffman defines in observing a person's actions as a performance in everyday life as 'the expression that he *gives*, and the expression that he *gives off'* (Goffman 1990: p. 14). As Lynch (2015) suggests, Goffman's notion gives us an insight into sympathetic presence and how we might identify it in person-centred leaders. For Lynch in this context and using Goffman's terms, sympathetic presence is identified when one *gives it*; it is a purposeful *showing* of a presence (p. 6–7). The findings of this study offer a crucial distinction in that what the 'audience', or for our example a patient, *gives off* deeply affects how the 'performer', or nurse, should *give* a presence back and vice versa. The findings suggest that sympathetic presence is an active performativity that relies on the inter-dependence of what is 'given' and what is 'given off' from both people in an interaction. The 'giving' and 'giving off' of sympathetic presence is an interplay, where one influences the other in a continuous cycle. It is, therefore, a dialogue. Understanding sympathetic presence through performativity represents both this and the potential that performance practice has in developing an understanding of and articulation of sympathetic presence.

The group demonstrated an understanding of how communication involves both verbal and non-verbal elements. They also showed an awareness that communicating sympathetically relies on intention, clarity, and context, and identified the role body language has in communicating sympathy beyond words.

> *Hannah: I think your body language –*
>   *Jamie: yeah*
>   *Rowan: aye*
>   *Hannah: it's more than your verbals when you're being sympathetic* (Focus Group: 364–367)

What the drama course revealed was that this same process of understanding personhood in others and oneself could be done in increasingly abstract ways whilst remaining alive and practical. For instance, the use of applied puppetry with 'person-less' objects facilitated the participant's understanding of interaction and presence as well as helped them practice applying their new understanding of personhood through sympathetic presence. The participants found the medical mannequins the most useful objects when exploring object theatre and applied puppetry. Some reported that this was due to their utility and approximation of human features, suggesting that there are limits to the level of abstraction. However, the fact these objects were not human had a significant effect. As Wiame asserts in her work into puppetry and Deleuzian philosophy, though some can look like humans it is always clear that 'puppets actually are not, and thus can help embrace a thought in which human beings are not at the centrum' (2016: p. 65). This displacement of centrality can become a key part of this approach concerning how performing sympathetic presence contributes to dignifying the distinct personhoods of others, particularly when they become increasingly abstracted from our dominant notion of 'the human'. There is much work to unveil the distinctions between what we mean when we say 'human', and 'person'. My doctoral study and this book as a whole, have put these terms alongside nursing and drama, raising questions on how we perform care with, through, and for materiality, and pointedly how this informs drama-based approaches to educate person-centred nurses.

The use of puppetry with mannequins and objects in the course enhanced certain elements of the participants' learning regarding communication. Using mannequins as simulated patients in role plays and short improvisations had particularly interesting results in this research study. Firstly, the lack of verbal communication from the mannequin meant that the participants had to pay closer attention to the details of what these mannequins were trying to express without the use of words. Reid-Searl et al. (2014) describe their approach *Pup-Ed*, where tutors animate puppets as patients in an SRP. They suggest puppets can 'be an effective tool to improve the communication skills of nursing students in a simulation learning context' (Ibid: p. 1202). The findings from my study concur and point to an enhanced understanding of non-verbal communication as a key feature of applying puppetry to healthcare SRP.

According to Brodzinski in her wide-ranging study of how theatre relates to health, a focus on inter-professional dialogue in healthcare environments can often mean the patient's 'voice is actually drowned out' (2010: p. 92). The mannequins used in the course were left silent to simulate this very issue, as well as others such as patients being non-verbal after a recent stroke, when they are in shock, and so on. Meanwhile, the participants were tasked with including the mannequins in the inter-action despite the mannequin's silence. As reported by Tizzard-Kleister and Jennings (2020), using mannequins can increase the difficulty of developing and demonstrating person-centred communication skills. It does this by abstracting the person at the centre and making communication with them 'non-natural'. The students cannot just rely on their natural and instinctive approaches, they must examine them, understand them, and then purposefully use them with a non-human person. At a deeper level, they must actively perform person-centredness to help bring the personhood of the puppet to life. Applying drama techniques such as those explored in this study seems to help. The group discovered how the acting techniques learnt through the drama-based exercises could be applied to their interactions with the mannequins. As a result, this showed how one can simulate a person-centred and caring exchange with them as well as you might a human-standardised patient. This is a strong example of the adaptability of the drama-based approach as an easily repeatable and potentially technical approach to teaching these skills.

The group reported how taking part in the process of puppetry—and actively respecting different objects—could help them relate to a 'patient' who cannot reply verbally. The notion of considering an object as a person was strange for many, but the value of the exercises was fairly clear for the group. This value was linked to the treatment of objects and the treatment of people, suggesting puppets/objects can help us to understand that respect and care can be performed for anyone—or indeed anything. This suggested that the techniques and understandings being developed by the group in this course are adaptable to many different situations, and many different people.

• *I could see and understand why we animated puppets to be like people, although they are non-living objects, but I value how respect can be shown to everyone and everything!* (Nic: 492–494)

In this context, the impossibility of one person fully understanding another's perspective became clear when a non-human took the place of a person in this exchange. This use of objects also evokes the critique of conventional notions of empathy, highlighting the impossibility of truly feeling what others are feeling. What does a plastic and rubber mannequin feel after all? Perhaps the mannequin's effectiveness stems from them being close, but not too close, to looking human. This arguably exposes a vital aspect of sympathetic presence, which involves a recognition of the distinctiveness of the other and a receptiveness to that difference.

The use of applied puppetry provided the participants with opportunities to perform sympathetic presence with objects *as if* they were human patients. This relates to— as Reeves et al. (2021) highlight in their study on drama, nursing, and empathy—how Rogers understood empathy as an imagined 'what if'. It is from this position that Rogers developed person-centredness, where the individual cannot assume they share the same feelings as others, but might imagine them. Applying these ideas to the concept of sympathetic presence through the translational and imagination-based process of applied puppetry (Smith 2015; Tizzard-Kleister and Jennings 2020) helped the participants in the course to discover a practical and embodied understanding of sympathetic presence through an abstract and simulated experience. Moreover, this experience showed how sympathetic presence helps to show respect and care for those one interacts with through an active and practical performativity of that presence.

The ability to engage with sympathetic presence in an abstract situation served to sharpen the participants' focus on how to do the same in other situations. Moreover, the participants found and believed that if they could respect and care for a collection of sticks animated by the entire cohort as an abstract simulated patient, they could perform the same respect and care for any person in any situation using similar techniques. In other words, they saw care as a relationship. Drama-based activity provided these burgeoning nurses a variety of opportunities to practice this performance of care. Drama also offers a tentative practical interactive 'vocabulary' in which to enhance this through practice, often through what is called 'performativity'. For example, the techniques from the drama course appeared to influence how the participants engaged in performing care in their practice learning. I suggest that the drama course, and the learning on sympathetic presence within the course, made a difference to how the participants performed care.

> *Gabrielle: you have to act as if they're there, and they were just talking over him. And I just remember thinking, oh my God that's horrible, that man can hear.*
> *Rowan: Aye.*
> *Gabrielle: He can – he was aware, he could move his side, but he just couldn't speak and they were speaking over him and I thought, nawh, that's not what I wanna do like. Yeah.*
> (Focus group: 1227–1233)

The ability to understand others through experience extended into a value system for Gabrielle's encounter with, and performance of care for, a non-verbal and non-mobile patient during her clinical placement. Gabrielle observed the lack of interaction given to this individual by her colleagues and by referring to her developed ideas on non-verbal communication and presence from the drama course cited a moral and ethical impulse to not repeat her colleague's actions. This reported incident shows how performing presence can directly communicate sympathy and ensure that care is person-centred through recognising the distinctiveness of the other and remaining open to them. It also shows that though this performance thrives on action and reaction (as all good drama does) the application of drama techniques bolstered the ability to perform these actions without obvious reactions from a patient. It could be said that the drama course enhanced the participant's 'response-ability'—to borrow Haraway's (2008) terms—and performativity. This suggests that for Gabrielle, and perhaps also for the other participants when and if they encounter similar situations, interacting sympathetically became easier, even without words and in many different situations, not least with less verbally active patients. Gabrielle maintained communication with her patient, remembering to at all times remain clear, effective, compassionate, and present. She achieved this by simply attending to him.

Conclusion

This chapter has presented the theme of 'attending to others'. Perhaps more so than the other main themes of this research study, this one represents something of a cycle the participants experienced at various points and in various configurations throughout the course. What this means is that the group discovered that by paying more attention to others, they found it easier to engage with them (including emotionally), leading to enhanced person-centred communication, which then feeds back into skills helping them to pay attention to others, and so on. This chapter presents the complementary development and symbiosis between drama-based activities and approaches to learning and person-centred nursing as a conceptual framework, and—more immediately—as a practice.

The next chapter, the last thematic chapter presents the final main theme, 'performing presence'.

References

Arrighi G, Irvine C, Joyce B, Kristi Haracz K (2018) Reimagining 'role' and 'character': an approach to acting training for role-play simulation in the tertiary education setting. Appl Theatre Res 6(2):89–106

Arveklev SH, Wigert H, Berg L, Burton B, Lepp M (2015) The use and application of drama in nursing education—an integrative review of the literature. Nurse Educ Today 35(7):E12–E17

Arveklev SH, Berg L, Wigert H, Morrison-Helme M, Lepp M (2018) Nursing students experiences of learning about nursing through drama. Nurse Educ Pract 28:60–65

Berardi F (2015) And: phenomenology of the end. Semiotext(e), South Pasadena

Boal A (1998) Theatre of the oppressed. Pluto Press, London

Brodzinski E (2010) Theatre in health and care. Palgrave, Basingstoke

Doolen J, Mariani B, Atz T, Horsley TL, Rourke JO, McAfee K, Cross CL (2016) High-fidelity simulation in undergraduate nursing education: a review of simulation reviews. Clin Simul Nurs 12(7):290–302

Ekebergh M, Lepp M, Dahlberg K (2004) Reflective learning with Drama in nursing education—a Swedish attempt to overcome the theory praxis gap. Nurse Educ Today 24:622–628

Goffman E (1990) The presentation of self in everyday life. Penguin, London

Haraway D (2008) When species meet. University of Minnesota Press, Minneapolis

Haraway D (2016) Staying with the trouble: making kin in the Chthulucene. Duke University Press, Durham

Hojat M (2009) Empathy in patient care: antecedents, development, measurement, and outcomes. Springer, New York

Kontos PC, Mitchell G, Mistry B, Ballon B (2010) Using drama to improve person-centred dementia care. Int J Older People Nursing 5(2):159–168

Lepp M (2002) Reflections on drama in nursing education in Sweden. Appl Theatre Res 3:1–6

Lieshout F, Cardiff S (2015) Reflections on being and becoming a person-centred facilitator. Int Pract Dev J 5. Available from: https://www.fons.org/library/journal/volume5-person-centredness-suppl/article4. Accessed 9 Mar 2018

Lynch B (2015) Partnering for performance in situational leadership: a person-centred leadership approach. Int Pract Dev J 5. Available from: https://www.fons.org/library/journal/volume5-person-centredness-suppl/article5. Accessed 13 Mar 2018

McAllister M, Reid-Searl K, Davis S (2013) Who is that masked educator? Deconstructing the teaching and learning processes of an innovative humanistic simulation technique. Nurse Educ Today 33(12):1453–1458

McCormack B, McCance T (2010) Person-centred nursing: theory and practice. Wiley-Blackwell, Chichester

Monden KR, Gentry L, Cox TR (2016) Delivering bad news to patients. Bayl Univ Med Cent Proc 29(1):101–102

Nursing and Midwifery Council (NMC) (2018) Future nurse: standards for proficiency and practice for registered nurses. NMC. Available from: future-nurse-proficiencies.pdf (nmc.org.uk). Accessed 1 June 2021

Nolan C (2009) Agency and embodiment: performing gestures/producing cultures. Harvard University Press, Harvard

Preston S (2016) Applied theatre: facilitation: pedagogies, practices, resistance. Bloomsbury Methuen, London

Reeves A, Neilson S (2018) 'Don't talk like that: It's not just what you say but how you say it': the process of developing an applied theatre performance to teach undergraduate nursing students communication skills around paediatric end-of-life care. J Appl Arts Health 9(1):99–111

Reeves A, Nyatanga B, Neilsen S (2021) Transforming empathy to empathetic practice amongst nursing and drama students. Res Drama Educ 26(2):1–18

Reid-Searl K, Mcallister M, Dwyer T, Krebs K, Anderson C, Quinney L, McLellan S (2014) Little people, big lessons: an innovative strategy to develop interpersonal skills in undergraduate nursing students. Nurse Educ Today 34:1201–1206

Simplican S (2015) Care, disability, and violence: theorizing complex dependency in Eva Kittay and Judith Butler. Hypatia 30(1):217–233

Skovdahl K, Dewing J (2017) Co-creating flourishing research practices through person-centred research: a focus on persons living with dementia. In: McCormack B, Dulmen S, Eide H, Skovdahl K (eds) Person-Centred healthcare research. Wiley-Blackwell, Chichester, pp 85–94

Sloan C (2018) Understanding spaces of potentiality in applied theatre. Res Drama Educ. The Journal of Applied Theatre and Performance 23(4):582–597

Smith M (2015) The practice of applied puppetry: antecedents and tropes. Res Drama Educ: The Journal of Applied Theatre and Performance 20(4):531–536

Tait P (2021) Theory for theatre studies: emotion. Methuen Drama, London

Tizzard-Kleister K, Jennings M (2020) "Breath, belief, focus, touch": applied puppetry in simulated role play for person-centred nursing education. Appl Theatre Res 8(1):73–87

White M (2009) Arts development in community health: a social tonic. Radcliffe, Oxford

Wiame A (2016) Deleuze's 'puppetry' and the ethics of non-human compositions. Maska 31(179/190):60–67

Performing Presence

8

Introduction

This chapter brings Part 2 to a close and is the final act in the story of my doctoral studies and the journey I have undertaken to explore how drama can be applied to person-centred nursing education. As with the previous three chapters, this one attends to one of the main themes from the analysis of the data collected from my doctoral study. This final theme 'performing presence' shows how the participants combined aspects of each previous theme and how these are used in combination to better perform caring roles through consciously adapting how they performed their presence. Learning how to be more present at a given moment and feeling presence as a relationship between people in simulated role plays contextualised the drama-based activity into nursing situations. Techniques helped participants develop how they performed presence and different caring roles. The group explored how to navigate complex relationships and create and maintain a sympathetic presence shared between people in a mutual environment. This theme summates the findings of the study by illustrating how participants experienced sympathetic presence in multiple roles through drama-based activity—enhancing their understanding of the concept, and their ability to perform presence with others.

In many ways, this chapter and the theme it explores is the summation of each of the other themes as well as the underpinning theme of the study overall. This chapter presents and discusses how the participants understood the notion of authenticity through the combined prisms of drama-based practice, actor training, and person-centred nursing. This is a prism where authenticity is found within the commitment to the actions offered and in the engagement of the personhood of a person with another. In a very connected sense, sympathetic presence is vital to this throughout. The participants discovered this through consistently feeling and practising sympathetic presence in different situations. This variety of circumstances helped the group to explore how sympathetic presence can be a starting point from which to build the role of the person-centred nurse. Not only did the repeated performance of

© The Author(s), under exclusive license to Springer Nature
Switzerland AG 2024
K. Tizzard-Kleister, *Applied Drama and Person-Centred Nursing*,
https://doi.org/10.1007/978-3-031-77208-5_8

this role centralise the notion of sympathetic presence as a key process to PCN, but these experiences evidenced that sympathetic presence is performative. What this notion relied on was seeing an authentic engagement at a given moment as a priority.

Being Authentically Present in the Moment

During the drama activities, the participants expressed that they felt like they were present at the moment and able to focus on what was happening around them. Drama activities seemed to promote paying attention to the present moment. Certain activities in the course prompted deep focus and attention.

> Jamie: And we did, in the drama we did, we just took time and I think at one stage we were like laying on the floor and being silent and pausing and thinking what's going on just right now – (Focus group: 1335–1339)

The group also explored how one's level of engagement must be relative to the situation and persons involved in a situation. They also explored how the affective quality of 'engagement' comes from the generosity with which this engagement is offered. McCormack and McCance (2010) also caution that one can go too far and over or under-engage, suggesting a nuanced and conscious level of engagement is critical for person-centred nursing. The key difficulty identified through this study is that when one engages more with the technical work of nursing than they do the emotional work, their performance of sympathetic presence is disjointed and indistinct. The participants developed an ability to engage with others with as much or more attention as they gave to completing their technical tasks. They soon discovered that this was the first step in being better able to perform sympathetic presence. A final revelation was that sympathetic presence is possible whilst performing other technical tasks, though this is a difficult balancing act.

This lends weight to the suggestion in the theoretical framework in Part 1 that linked engagement and sympathetic presence through the work on applied drama facilitation by Preston (2016). Specifically, this is the notion that sympathetic presence is a negotiation of presented selves through a performed presence characterised by sympathy, whilst engagement is the generosity with which one offers themselves to an interaction. The results of my research study suggest that the drama-based activity encouraged student nurses to engage with and pay attention to their patients in the midst of completing technical tasks more effectively, enhancing and enhanced by their performance of sympathetic presence. This also served to highlight how, when a group of people collectively engage generously, a feeling akin to sympathetic presence permeates the environment. As it did when the group engaged with the 'slow walks' task where there was a group focus on sequential tasks which had undeniable aesthetic qualities, or the 'safe space' task where the group openly discussed emotionally complex feelings with generosity and conviviality.

Through purposefully using stasis and contemplation participants had more focus and felt able to pause and contemplate during and after action. In simple terms, the group explored being less immediately reactive to being thoughtfully responsive. Participants appeared better equipped to engage in contemplation along with other concurrent tasks, including paying attention to others such as simulated patients. This was at odds with the assumption that contemplative practice and pausing lead to stasis, or introspection to the point of inactivity.

Responses to this exercise focused on its hypnotic effect, many noting the intense focus required of the exercise. (Field notes: 416–418)

By performing sympathetic presence, the participants better recognised the personhood presented by others. Meanwhile, they attended to the authenticity of aspects of that presented personhood through that recognition. A study conducted by de Oliveira et al. (2015) looks at how drama can be used to enhance the psychological fidelity of an SRP and how using drama techniques in SRP might lead to more active attention from the participants. My finding is similar and shows how drama used effectively in SRP can enhance attention to the 'authentic' aspects of a simulation for the participant regardless of how high-tech a simulation suite is. Through the interactive role plays and drama-based activities, the participants experienced what performing a fixed presence feels like, such as an exercise where two people play nurses who are only allowed to talk to each other and must ignore a patient who is trying to get their attention without words. This showed how being unresponsive in one's presence often leads to stilted interactions and a feeling of inauthenticity from the person performing this static role. This challenged the assumption that authenticity is linked to a static self with unshakable moral certainty and immutable righteous virtue. This perception of personhood revealed through performing sympathetic presence is not one of individual truths and virtues, but of features, traits, and beliefs that contribute to a person's personhood in a given moment, whilst co-constructing a relationship with those they encounter. In this way, the concept of 'authenticity' is a constructed recognition and validation of what is authentic in a given moment and between people, rather than an essentialist truth or an absolute moral imperative.

However, unlike personhood understood through performing sympathetic presence, 'authenticity' is not entirely co-constructed. Rather, as the participants soon realised, authentic (or perhaps 'truthful' is the better term here) traits are easier to identify through the language of sensation and sympathy activated by sympathetic presence than, say, verbal exchanges between people who do not engage with one another. For instance, the group attested to how it is easier to *feel* if someone is in pain even if they deny that they are, by attuning to them through sympathetic presence. In this way, they are attending to their authentic sensations through sympathetic presence. This resonated with how the participants saw the drama-based activity and simulation learning as useful learning through trying out different roles, which directly related to their future practice. These activities, and the perceptions and feelings which grew from engaging in them, were both individually effective and noticeable in a group dynamic. The seeming simplicity of some tasks, such as walking as slowly as possible with certain actions and internalisations, was both enjoyable and challenging for the group. These types of exercises promoted an awareness of both the world around the participants and the imagined experience of those who embody similar ways of moving—such as those with difficulties walking as Alice reflected.

I enjoyed the chair exercise! Being focused to remember to walk slowly made me feel how it must feel for someone who can't walk. (Alice: 36–37)

This finding concurs with Maurice Hamington's assertion that '[a]n authentically caring performance is one that can adapt to the circumstances with deft enquiry and responsive action' (2020: p. 33). The participants demonstrated this and highlighted the importance of sensations and feelings in doing so. The results of my research study show that by engaging in drama-based activity and SRP for a longer duration the participants were better able to understand and pay attention to personhood as an expression of an individual's authenticity in that moment through performing sympathetic presence.

Throughout the drama course, the participants began to see how engaging in and applying acting techniques enhanced their simulations. In some circumstances, these techniques provided a method of thinking through and improving their real-life interactions with others. The consideration that these approaches promote inauthentic feelings and emotions became less of a concern as the participants understood that every interaction could be understood as a performance. Returning to Preston (2016), these terms applied to what can be called a facilitative practice can cause difficulties in how one perceives oneself. However, to move away from the limiting concern of whether one is being authentic or inauthentic, the drama course focused on how one could actively perform actions that are 'constantly performative and responsive', fostering 'critical reflexivity which monitors and *notices* rather than moralises about the impact on the self' (Preston 2016: p. 48). For instance, the group could see how the authenticity of a particular action could be better characterised by how well it helped to achieve a caring objective and how it felt as an intention characterised by compassion, and less how it aligned with their 'authentic personhood'.

More precisely, the authenticity of an interaction lay in pursuing a caring objective which actively responded and attended to the personhood of the 'cared for' other, rather than trying to reinforce their perceptions of themselves. Though the group began to see the drama-based approach as useful in this way, they were hesitant to use this terminology regarding patients. They could see how acting techniques might be used to enhance their communication and ability to perform presence, but it was less clear to them how this may apply to helping them understand the behaviour of others. Understandably, the participants did not want to diminish the feelings, experiences, or responses of their 'real' patients as people—particularly people who might be bioethically vulnerable or endangered. Upon reflection, it may have been useful to use the ideas of actor training to consider and analyse how others might be subconsciously and consciously using different actions and objectives in everyday scenarios in more depth.

The exploration of what may inhibit an individual from engaging fully with the interaction at hand, or becoming more present in that moment, was also reported on. For example, participants displayed and identified moments of overthinking and tension as things getting in the way of enhancing their performance. Some exercises highlighted the need to lessen tensions caused by overthinking and to recognise this tension as a barrier to being present.

> *I could do it better if I stopped overthinking it.*
> *However I think I did good - it's a learning process.* (Jamie: 720–721)

Through taking part in the course, the group confirmed feeling sympathetic presence as a result of certain activities as well as demonstrating an understanding that one can perform precise and practised presences. This shifted their understanding of the concept of presence as a passive to an active state, from a state of 'being' and into a performed 'doing'. This therefore suggests that understanding sympathetic presence as a shared feeling is more accessible and useful in early PCN education. I argue that the participants could feel, create, and sustain sympathetic presence in what could be described as a simulated and performative environment. As a result, it is wholly possible to simulate sympathetic presence.

Whilst engaging with this shift in perspective the notion of acting and drama-based activity as 'faking it' rather than truly feeling sympathetic presence was challenged. In a related way to how sympathetic presence seen as performative helps to find authenticity in a given moment as discussed above, the application of actor training techniques also helps to make sense of the authenticity of 'performed' feelings and emotions. Actor training gives a process for nursing students to perform different roles, combining this approach with the concepts and practices of PCN leads us towards an understanding that these roles are constructed, authentic in their application, and pragmatic to actualise person-centred care. Preston (2016) highlights a similar experience for applied drama facilitators who feel they are manufacturing emotions in their practice. Preston explains that for these facilitators '[m]oving between roles that feel authentic and inauthentic cannot always easily be reconciled and can create dissonant feelings that are difficult to manage' (p. 48). This is crucial for both nursing and applied drama facilitation as both depend on practitioners who are open and responsive as well as in a good place in themselves to better care for others. It could be stated that both applied drama facilitators and nurses must perform different 'selves' to suit different situations, with a focus on facilitating and caring for others more effectively. I argue that applied drama facilitators might benefit from learning more about actor training just as the nursing students in my study have. By doing so, they may be able to apply the practice as a way of accessing 'inauthentic' roles with greater comfort and success, whilst reconciling the potential ill effects of guilt at not being authentic and ultimately, empathetic. Both professions could certainly benefit from re-balancing 'affective' and 'cognitive' empathy, to avoid over-arousal, armouring up, and burnout (Heggestad et al. 2016).

As Lieshout and Cardiff (2015) report '[o]nce we start to combine being person-centred with facilitation, a specific type of relationship emerges where connectedness and reciprocity foster mutual growth' (p. 3). Clearly, focusing attention on one's concerns is a barrier to effectively considering and responding to others, but ignoring them entirely is equally stultifying. By including ideas around facilitation practice, specifically applied drama influenced 'critical facilitation' (Preston 2016), the drama course offered the participants a way to improve their performance of presence and understand their role in that. Furthermore, the participants learnt that sympathetic presence as a performative process is always active. By confirming both Preston's (2016) and Lieshout and Cardiff's (2015) arguments, my research study suggests that the drama-based practice facilitates participants to better deal with feelings of 'faking it' and to engage and connect with others with sympathetic presence.

Certain exercises brought up feelings of presence, promoting learning and exploration about presence as something to feel between people in a given moment. Silence and pausing served to heighten the groups' awareness of this feeling. Initially, participants responded warily to questions like 'Did you feel that?' However, they were quick to agree that they felt *something* in these moments. Morgan in particular described feeling the presence of others in the group around her more acutely as a result of the activities in the course.

> At the end of the cycle a silence falls over the group, which Matt purposefully does not fill. There are giggles and unsurety. Matt then explains that there is a feeling in the room, asking participants what this is. I've noted he asks "Do you feel that?" The participants who speak up agree that there is some feeling present. Morgan in particular notes that she feels as if she can feel the group around them. For Matt, this is spot on. This, it is described, is presence. (Field notes: 139–145)

Feeling and Practising Sympathetic Presence

Demonstrably, the group were able to identify when interactions were not sympathetic, and when the presence of others was lacking in sympathy. They were best able to do this in the role of the patient who directly experienced the presence of their peers who were performing as nurses. They were able to give feedback to their peers on their feelings and experiences during the role play. This demonstrates the participants' enhanced embodied knowledge about sympathetic presence. This suggests that these embodied experiences which gave the participants some access to the experiences of others enhanced their understanding of sympathetic presence through an ability to embody it. I argue that when sympathetic presence is approached from a chiefly theoretical standpoint it remains an abstract and often unachievable novelty, which only very few people are innately able to 'do'. The drama course, and how it has affected the participant's abilities, clearly shows that sympathetic presence is something enacted and felt between people. It is not within one person and it is not a trait, rather it is a nuanced and sensitive performance which is enhanced through both theoretical and practical applications. This means that 'understanding' it requires experience from both theoretical and practical standpoints—knowing it theoretically doesn't mean one can 'do it', whilst being able to 'do it' without knowing why or how means it might not be done as effectively. This is a particular highlight of the research study's findings, offering a key insight into the concept of sympathetic presence through the use of drama-based activity. It was evident that the group felt something, though they could not define this feeling as clearly as they would have liked and had to rely on more general terms rather than ideas from the course, or their nursing degree, such as sympathetic presence. Other activities led participants to feel an increased awareness of the presence of others as well as a deeper understanding of personal space.

In many of our discussions after this particular exercise participants frequently refer to personal space and feeling the presence of the others around them. (Field notes: 202–204)

This study's findings suggest that the discovery around sympathetic presence directly relates to an understanding of personhood, namely that it too is performative, and performed in relational with the personhood of others in a given moment. The scenarios explored through the SRP and other drama-based activities highlighted the fact that patients often do not act as one might wish them to, nor are nurses immune to the feelings of those they work with. In this way, participants developed an ability to recognise the personhood of others through actively recognising and attending to differences between themselves and others. In turn, this highlighted the criticality of remaining open to others to be better able to recognise their personhood.

This challenges one aspect of Kitwood's definition of personhood, namely how personhood can be considered as 'a standing or status that is bestowed upon one human being, by others, in the context of relationship and social being' (1997: p. 8). Instead, the participants expressed an understanding that though personhood is indeed relational in a given moment, it is not bestowed by one to another but co-constructed by each person in the interaction. This is clear to see in the group's early focus on notions of selfhood as opposed to personhood, explored in Chap. 5. By interacting with others in various shifting roles, they discovered how much of that role, or self, is constructed by other people in that moment. Lieshout and Cardiff (2015) describe personhood as a constant state of becoming which characterises the personhood of an individual, who 'in relation create[s] social structures, conventions and practices which in turn influence their being (in relation)' (p. 5). In contrast to Kitwood's definition, this does not mean one person bestows personhood onto another, but that each person's personhood is defined through distinction with—and in relationship to—others. It is therefore argued with the support of the findings of this study that personhood is understood and created through relationality, based on identifying differences.

These interactions with others in different and changing roles led to the group feeling what they agreed felt like sympathetic presence, particularly during the role-play exercises. Participants were able to identify these feelings as what sympathetic presence might feel like through engaging with and paying attention to others and their surroundings at that moment. Even in the simulated environment, participants were reportedly able to create, sustain, and feel this in practice. They suggest that this feeling leads to more awareness of the situation and a heightened sense of the presence of others.

> Rowan: I think whenever we done that there – I played the family member, and yous were [To Nic and Hannah] the doctors and nurses.
>> Karl: [to Hannah] the one that Hannah really didn't like! [laughter]
>> Hannah: haha, no
>> Rowan: I felt that then, I thought.
>> Jamie: yeah, I agree. (Focus group: 556–563)

The course offered the experience of what interacting with others in a variety of performed roles may feel like. This enhanced the depth of perception each participant had of themselves and others. This tapped into what MacNeill et al. (2016) highlight in their study on healthcare staff using drama to develop their role, as learning which is 'not primarily conceptual but rather perceptual' (p. 210). MacNeill et al.'s research highlights the potential to engage in multiple forms of understanding through drama-based activity, which the findings of this study support. For instance, how the participants could immediately and unanimously feel 'something like' sympathetic presence through perception but struggled to articulate what sympathetic presence is as a cognitive exercise. The drama-based approach also allowed interjections, the application of techniques and the ability to re-attempt a scenario in a new role, with a new understanding of the self. As MacNeill et al. state, drama-based techniques and acting applied to professional healthcare are about 'playing one's role more effectively' (Ibid: p. 210).

Building on this sentiment, the findings of this study suggest that there is no one role, no singular 'knowing self' or singular attribute definable as a 'prerequisite' which perfectly suits any given situation. As McCormack and McCance (2010) discuss, the 'knowing self' recognises what one *does not know* and should be characterised by openness and relationality. I argue that response-ability, metaphorical translations, speaking the language of sensibility, and generosity also characterise a 'knowing self', as evidenced by the conceptual frame in Part 1, and the research findings in Part 2. McCormack & McCance draw on Schön's (1983) idea of 'reflecting on action' as a way of engaging 'in a process of continuous learning' towards 'professional practice' (McCormack and McCance 2010: p. 59). As Arveklev et al. (2020) argues, Schön's idea of 'reflection on action', where one reflects on something after it has happened, has become a dominant method in nursing pedagogy. Whereas the less considered partner idea of 'reflecting in action' (where one reflects and reacts at the moment) offers 'an ability that is crucial when tackling complex situations in nursing care' (p. 5). The findings of this research study concur with both McCormack and McCance (2010) and Arveklev et al. (2020) and argues that drama offers a compelling pedagogical approach for developing practitioners' abilities to reflect both in and on action to in turn develop an open and relational 'knowing self' when performing sympathetic presence. Moreover, this is a knowing self with greater acuity in response-ability, metaphorical translation, the language of sensibility, and generosity.

To be precise, there is no singular way to perform sympathetic presence, it is not *a* performance, it is a mode of *performativity*. As such, the role of the person-centred nurse should therefore be fluid, relational, and responsive. This adaptability is a skill which can be enhanced through drama-based activity. It is evident that the participants in this research course played their person-centred roles more effectively as a result of the drama-based activity through performing sympathetic presence which was responsive to the situation and persons involved. Participants felt that the adaptable techniques they learnt were useful in being present and directly helping those they cared for. These techniques, and their skilled and contextual use, were directly linked to enhancing the participants' ability to help others.

> *[...]powerful tool to be using to help others in my care.* (Alice: 176–177)

However, participants mostly identified generalised approaches from the learning, rather than specific methods, for example, how to read body language and identify what others might be trying to present and communicate. It was through these approaches that the participants seemed to develop a better understanding of how a specific person communicates. Though particular ways of achieving this were not mentioned, it is stated that engaging with the drama and applying this learning aided in doing so.

> *Rowan: Yeah, I thought that like from the drama, just reading someone's persona-*
> *Gabrielle: Body language.*
> *Rowan: Body language, or eye contact, you just knew, what way they wanted to communicate.* (Focus Group: 1200–1204)

Although specific methods such as 'actions' and 'objectives' were mentioned and explained during the course and had an observable effect on the participants' performance within the role plays, they were not remembered terminologically. However, the ability to apply them to interaction was both observed and reported to improve both the role play and interactions in practice learning environments. This was particularly noticeable in 'non-clinical', everyday, interactions with patients, showing an appreciation for, and ability to, interact more confidently and effectively. This is the opposite effect of the highlighted issue with teaching the 6 C's (Lawrence and Wier 2018). In the case of the 6 C's students can recite them, but there it is less clear how they apply them to their practice or what they mean. In our case, the application to practice is felt and expressed by the participants, and observable, whilst they are less able to recite the techniques and/or ideas terminologically. What this suggests is that the approach of the drama course led to higher levels of learning based on Bloom's Taxonomy (1956), where 'remembering' the information was less important than 'applying' and 'synthesising' it.

Interestingly, Nic reports how his confidence in interacting was enhanced, and also that the drama led to him treating 'every patient the same'. Though this could be interpreted to suggest that the drama encouraged the delivery of homogenous and mechanistic care, where interactions with patients are identical and most definitely not person-centred, Nic's inference here is an equality of respect and attention.

> *Nic: Before that she says I'd rather stay at home and not come in for the treatments. But the nurses, she says, really did help for sorta me coming and getting my treatment. She says the fact you come in and you ask me how am I and how are things with you today, she says it really does make a difference she says, I couldn't' – you're gunna be a great nurse in the future and wished me the very best and uh – but it's only through the drama, that I'd have treated every patient the same, treat no patient differently.* (Focus Group: 1107–1113)

Learning these techniques in a simulated environment meant that the learning was perceived as highly adaptable and relatable and seemed to prepare the group for future situations. It was suggested that the course prompted participants to re-apply the performance approaches they explored in the course to achieve more equal and consistently compassionate interactions. It was also clear that participants were far more confident with and able to engage in similar training activities outside of the course. For example, Gabrielle and Rowan both decided to take part as patient actors in the annual Community Resilience and Disaster Response exercise held at UU. This 1-day exercise involves teams of third-year nursing students taking part in role plays facilitated by emergency response organisations such as The Red Cross, members of the Police Service of Northern Ireland, the Ambulance Service and so on. Third year Nursing students undertake these role plays, which include a wide variety of siulated situations where emergency care is needed such as terrorists attacks, drug-related incidents, chemical accidents, and more. The students are assessed on their ability to navigate these challenging scenarios. First- and second-year nursing students (as the participants of my study were at the time) are invited to take part as patient actors in these scenarios. Reportedly, both Gabrielle and Rowan found these role plays easier to take part in due to their participation in the course.

> *Gabrielle: Well there shouldn't really be a difference, because – well it did at the start, at the start when we were doing the role plays I felt a wee bit funny, but like coming in to do that day with Pat, it was like an actual thing, because you'd been –*
> *Rowan: Because you'd already done the drama here.* (Focus group: 1356–1366)

It appeared to be the variety of increasingly complex activities, including SRP, that helped to promote an escalating understanding of how to perform a certain presence. In this case, the group explored a specific presence that characterises a person-centred nurse. This specific presence was discovered to be analogous to sympathetic presence.

Exploring and Performing the Role of the Person-Centred Nurse through Sympathetic Presence

The drama course highlighted how sympathetic presence should be performed as a crucial part of how a person-centred nurse presents themselves and interacts with others. Through the drama course, participants learnt how to consciously perform their presence using drama-based techniques such as playing 'actions'. They also learnt how this performance hinged on thinking in a person-centred way, where the perspectives of others were not assumed but recognised, respected, and responded to. It was crucial that the participants could pay attention to others, whilst simultaneously engaging with their own and other's emotional states. They came to understand that they might never fully understand the feelings or emotions of others, but they could nevertheless interact with them sensitively through sympathetic presence.

All of these ideas influenced how the participants came to understand the utility of performing a particular presence as a presentation of a self. This presentation of a self can be understood as a role or as Goffman puts it a 'front' (1990). To ensure one consistently and effectively performs sympathetic presence, this role—or 'front'—should be adaptive and responsive to the person and personhood of those involved in a given moment. The course served as a space to develop a practical ability to perform multiple roles more effectively. The application of drama-based practices gave participants a language and medium through which to adapt their performance in the activities explored in the drama course. This included techniques from Stanislavski's MoPA, such as using different 'actions' to achieve different 'objectives' (Stanislavski 1990; Benedetti 1998; Merlin 2014).

On a more fundamental level, the use of phrases like 'character', 'front', 'role', or 'show' by the participants when describing interacting with others made it clear that each interaction can be considered as a presentation of a particular self to achieve a specific objective. The participants were better able to recognise the importance of playing a particular role, and displayed an ability to consciously perform these roles in different circumstances. This is similar to Goffman's (1990) assertion that we perform roles in response to the social circumstance we are in different circumstances in his ethnographic studies of how people present themselves. Moreover, developing and modelling the performance of their role as a nurse was a method of 'dramatic realisation' for the participants. For Goffman, social activity is only made visible when it is realised or more precisely when it is actualised. In many cases, this requires a dramatic 'over-display' for the observer to recognise it. The drama course illustrated to the participants that it is necessary to enact—or rather to perform—sympathetic presence for it to be realised and felt.

Participants displayed an awareness of how you can develop techniques to improve how you might perform your role as a nurse as well as an awareness of how others perceive this performance and the effect performing different roles has on others. This directly relates to Goffman's concept of a front. Hannah observed how adapting your presence to suit the needs of the situation is vital as well as the use of the calming activities used in the drama course to achieve this.

Hannah: if you're with a patient and you have to calm them down, if you're going at all
nervous too, but I think if you do all that before that can calm you down as well, and you're
defusing the situation. (Focus Group: 16–18)

The findings of this study also suggest that it is important for the individual to
perform this dramatic realisation to deepen their 'knowing self', an identified prerequisite to PCN in the PCNF (McCormack and McCance 2010: p. 56–60).
Furthermore, the participants discovered that to have a lasting and meaningful
impression on patients and family members—to make them feel the care they
receive more acutely—the performances and caring work of the nurse should be
tactically emphasised 'to make it apparent that they are performing it well' (Goffman
1990: p. 43). This 'emphasis' does not necessarily need to be overt, but simply
points attention towards the actions performed by the nurse. It can be that a nurse
feels they are being sympathetic whilst a patient might not feel that is the case.
Although the nurse may think that their actions and words are conveying the sympathy, they intend them to, it is sometimes only by emphasising these actions and
words through a variety of interactive strategies that the sympathy which characterises them is 'dramatically realised'.[1] This relies on practitioners to consciously
adapt their presentation of self to make it easier for this sympathy to be felt by others. As such, understanding sympathetic presence as performative becomes an
important way in which nurses might develop and dramatically realise a knowing
self. By exploring and applying performance-based techniques as already discussed
(Stanislavski 1990; Boal 1998) the participants saw how their role as a nurse can be
adapted as part of a presentational and interactive skill set to actively and consciously achieve different caring outcomes.

Exercises and discussions provided a springboard to take a closer look at these
roles in various care contexts, including an exploration of the expected role that
nurses and patients traditionally play. Through exploring these roles participants
were able to question and challenge assumptions and encourage a shifted perspective of what role the nurse in particular can play, especially concerning the authority
given to them. Some activities tasked the group to use their position as a nurse to

---

[1] This is, I argue, a path for a powerful and simple way to communicate when considered in conjunction with Stanislavski's Objectives and Given Circumstances. For example, we might overemphasise an action performed to ensure it is "dramatically realised", likewise we might state and
affirm an objective we have, and even attempt to verbalise what we sense another person's objective might be, to communicate clearly and effectively. Giving a practical example, a nurse may say
to their patient, "I want you to remain in bed, but I sense you wish to get out of bed". This clarifies
what each person is trying to achieve from a nurse's perspective, the patient may correct the suggestion of what the nurse feels they want and has a better understanding of what the nurse is hoping
to achieve. This develops further when we add given circumstances. Continuing the example, the
nurse may say: "I want you to stay in bed, as if you get up you may reopen your wound, which
would be very dangerous for you, as well as distressing for me." This added context alongside a
clearly stated objective can be firm ground to start a meaningful dialogue. It may be, perhaps, that
the patient feels they must get up, regardless of the risk, and are now aware of the nurse's position,
they may then be able to negotiate and reach a shared decision. I will halt this example here, as it
should be clear already that applying these approaches to a situation is simple in approach, but
adds complexity very quickly.

influence others, using actions which made use of these roles in different ways, and to navigate the responsibility of that power and influence. This appeared to lead to Jamie's realisation that this position could easily be misused, and reportedly incited a deeper commitment to not allow this to happen.

Patients feel vulnerable - they see nurses as someone in a position of power - it's important not to get carried away - make them feel reassured and comfortable. (Jamie: 392–394)

Practical activities encouraged the group to explore ways of positively using their role as nurses in interactions with others, such as building trust and being reassuring. By focusing on relationships and interactions in SRPs, the group had opportunities to perform and adapt their roles to achieve their objectives whilst maintaining a sympathetic presence with others. These experiences raised issues of trust, comfort, and responsibility for others when working as a nurse. The sensation of losing control, or taking it, was expressed clearly by the participants as memorable and difficult, suggesting a deeper appreciation of how they might use their authority and ability to influence others to achieve certain outcomes. For example, Nic was playing a nurse during a role play with Alice as a patient. Alice felt her task was getting out of bed to get a drink; Nic was tasked with keeping Alice in her bed for her safety.

Nic tries to show Jamie that it is 2AM, saying "trust me, it's 2AM", which is an interesting attempt to use their own position of power to imply trust. (Field notes: 2146–2148)

The place of compassion in person-centred nursing is a nuanced one, and as the participants demonstrated, can be offset by a mechanistic approach to nursing. As de Zulueta (2013) explains through an examination of the place of compassion in healthcare in the twenty-first century, a focus on completing tasks creates a 'mechanistic' environment where healthcare staff struggle to be compassionate in the presence of others (p. 123). This is particularly relevant for the participants and their development of understanding person-centredness and sympathetic presence. Particularly so as both person-centredness and sympathetic presence draw deeply on compassionate communication.

As Hojat (2009) theorises, empathy and sympathy are overlapping processes and the point at which they meet lies compassion. It might be attractive to reconsider sympathetic presence as, say, 'compassionate presence', however, this balance between empathy and sympathy as described by Hojat is difficult to achieve in practice. McCormack & McCance remind us that '[o]ne cannot force someone to be caring' (2010: p. 83). More so, drawing on Kitson (1987), they remind us that compassion can be seen as an 'imperfect duty' that refers more to a 'moral attitude' based on 'the moral character of the individual' (McCormack and McCance 2010: p. 83). In contrast, sympathetic presence is an active process located in the relationships between people. As the participants discovered in the research course, sympathetic presence *can be compassionate*. However, it is not based on an impulse to care compassionately in every instance, recognising the impossibility of any person being able to perform this sensitive moral 'balancing act' at all times, for all people they encounter. In simple terms, it can be dispassionate if the situation demands it.

At its heart, it is a performed and pragmatic presence that seeks to provide what is needed by each person at a given moment. Sympathetic presence, as evidenced by the participants' ability to consciously perform it, allows the practitioner to be present and engaged, without the constant demands to maintain the 'moral attitude' of compassion as an 'imperfect duty', whilst also avoiding a 'mechanistic approach'. Moreover, continuing Hojat's (2009) thread, if empathy and sympathy are a continuum, we need more sympathy within nursing to offset the overuse of empathy in education and practice.

The practical activities in the drama course were often intended to challenge participants to assess their ability to assume various roles to achieve different care outcomes through performing sympathetic presence. Some of the group frequently distance themselves from their personal feelings, wearing their uniform like armour—as previously explored. They did this by playing the role of a nurse who is being overly distanced from their activities as well as playing the role of a patient who is interacting with that nurse. Experiencing this from both the perspective of a nurse and a patient links the feeling of hopelessness often felt by a patient, to the distancing performed by the nurse. The participants demonstrably developed their awareness and understanding of the effects of this tactic of distancing during these practical activities—along with many others. As a result, participants were able to identify how a distanced demeanour may negatively affect others, and how nurses might perform 'a front' that is not distanced but engaged for the benefit of those in their care. Crucially, they also *felt* the difference in care that is and is not distanced (or rather, engaged) as they played the role of patient.

> Gabrielle: it's like subconscious
> Nic: it's behaviour
> Gabrielle: you're learning that you have to put up - it is a front, like you are putting on a completely - even if you're having a crap day, you're still putting on that the you had a good day
> Rowan: you need to still smile, like. (Focus Group: 1487–1490)

They were also able to identify methods to manage how they presented themselves beyond simply looking like a nurse, to in turn better perform suitable caring roles. The recognition that these roles are performed, and the importance of consciously performing these roles—through the techniques and experiences from the course—was displayed by the participants. It emerged that concerns of inauthenticity about actor training and drama were perhaps misplaced and related to performing a nursing role more directly than the participants may have considered.

> Gabrielle: I think it's quite the same now. Looking back before we went out on placement, I'd be like, Nawh, but now, it is. [...] you're putting on a show, you're not, but you have to have this kind of way about you. (Focus group: 315–320)

The participants commented on how the variety of the situations presented through role plays and drama-based exercises made it clear that a singular scripted approach to interacting with others is not helpful. By engaging in an improvisational approach to caring interactions, the group were performing what Hamington defines as an 'improvisational moral performance'. This is where 'normativity, or the right thing to do, is understood as emergent within relational experience' (2020: p. 21, 22). The finding also confirms the hypothesis in Part 1 that applying elements of Stanislavski's MoPA might enhance a participant's ability to perform a future 'naturalism'. This is not a naturalism played out on the stage, rather it enhances how one can perform in everyday reality. The drama course highlighted how effective communication goes beyond scripted responses and the exclusivity of verbal language in every interaction.

Through the use of acting techniques, such as Stanislavskian 'actions', 'objectives', and 'given circumstances', participants saw how to mesh their objective with others to achieve mutual goals within a given situation. Goodwin and Deady (2013) describe the use of Stanislavskian actor training techniques within nursing education as 'allowing practitioners to enhance the levels of empathy they display' (p. 131). They argue that the use of 'emotional memory' is a key part of Stanislavski's system. They suggest that the use of emotion memory alongside the previously mentioned aspects of the MoPA helps build a nurse's '"bank" of sensory and (more importantly) emotional sensations' as well as helping them to 'develop the ability to deftly use these sensations to find common ground with clients' (Ibid: p. 132). The findings of my study challenge the need for emotion memory as a technique to access, understand, and perform emotionally challenging interactions. Focusing on the findings of this research study I argue against the use of 'emotional memory' because it leads to an over-exposure to—and static exploration of—sensitive feelings rather than an integration of an active ability to perform caring actions through enhanced responsive and interactive sensibility. I also contest the value and sustainability of relying on one's emotional memory to access empathy with another person's emotional state. The irony of using one's own emotions to try to understand the emotions of others is—I hope—clear. Instead, I advocate for using actor training to enhance one's ability to perform embodied sympathetic presence. Emotion memory may be suitable as a small part in 'rehearsing' this but is unhelpful in its performance. Just as Nolan (2009) describes the repeated motion of a graffiti artist inscribing paint onto the walls, and the movements inscribing knowledge into their body, it is the action that creates the meaning, not the memory. What this study adds, is that these actions need actualisation—or rather dramatic realisation (Goffman 1990), or even better yet, performing—and practice to be inscribed and embodied? Sympathetic presence *must* be practised as a performative skill. A focus on emotion memory in isolation from Stanislavski's other approaches is a worrying trend in collaborations between nursing and drama that continues to ask too much of people to draw on their reserves to discover emotional engagement with others. Asking someone to understand and feel the pain of another is debilitating. The use of the MoPA has provided the participants of the drama course with an active approach to performing sympathetically present care more aligned with Hamington's notion of an 'improvisational moral performance' (2020: p. 21) without continually drawing from their emotional reserves.

Sympathetic presence was seen by the group in my drama course as an atmosphere that could pervade a room as opposed to just a process that could be completed by an individual. The group identified that through engaging with many different drama-based exercises, a shared feeling and experience of what sympathetic presence might feel like was created and sustained. The group agreed that this required those in the room to be contributing to this feeling for it to work. This contribution required a synchronous individual and group effort, with the reported effect of the group feeling like they were 'at one'. This suggests an awareness of the relationship between the self and others and the importance of this relationship in performing sympathetic presence. Silence, focus, awareness of surroundings, and pausing seemed to be important factors in feeling and creating sympathetic presence. Again, participants were definitive in their agreement of this shared feeling and the change in the environment that it facilitates, but struggled to ascribe words to this sensation. Certain drama activities helped participants experience and subsequently become more aware of this feeling.

> *Karl: did you feel that room during that exercise had a sympathetic presence to it?*
> *[Talking over each other]*
> *Rowan: aye it felt like –*
> *Alice: yes –*
> *[...]*
> *Jamie: Oh, slow walk. It made you sort of like, pause or something. Dunno how, I'm trying to explain it. It definitely [...] I think that felt like sympathetic presence. Just like, being at one with – and Matt always said "I am me, and I am OK". I think that one too.*
> (Focus group: 425–429, 595–598)

Conclusion

This chapter has brought the presentation and discussion of the main findings of my doctoral study in context to the conceptual frame suggested in Part 1 to a conclusion. In these last four chapters, four main themes have been explored through presenting and discussing appropriate parts of the data that constructed them, with concepts from Part 1 and beyond fuelling the discussion on these findings.

This chapter has specifically looked at the main theme 'performing presence'. Though it can be said that all four of these themes are interwoven and mutually interdependent, the last of the themes more than any of the others represent the core of the central findings of this project. What this theme contributes is the fundamental necessity of a well-practised and well-performed sympathetic presence to the role of the person-centred nurse. In a broader sense, it has laid bare the great need for presence in nursing, and how drama can be a process and medium to encourage, develop, and access skills in performing that presence. This chapter also explores how the drama-based activities encouraged the experimentation and refinement of various performed presences for specific purposes. This chapter illustrated how the participants experienced something engaging in taking part in the course as well as discovering ways in which to engage in situations themselves with authenticity through the actions they performed with others. What was crucial in developing this was a greater acuity to feeling a presence, identifying whether this presence is sympathetic, and practising performing this presence. The participants helped to illuminate how the drama-based activities incited and greatly enhanced the performance of sympathetic presence. The culmination of this theme and chapter presents the interconnected link between performing sympathetic presence and the role of the person-centred nurse. I stand firm in arguing that this is a shared feature of nursing as a whole. Whether one calls it sympathetic presence or not, I suggest that this is something many nurses do, or have done. I am emboldened to state that it is the practice of this that defines nursing. Simply, nursing is actively being with others, and offering something which is sustaining, caring, and nourishing. Sympathetic presence, I conclude in this chapter and Part 2's arguments, is the atomised fundamental constituent of this *thing* nurses do.

These four chapters comprising Part 2 of this book have presented and discussed my doctoral research by highlighting the participants' contributions alongside concepts explored in Part 1. This represents the totality of the findings of my doctoral research. The next chapter offers some concluding thoughts, summarising the project's key features (including limitations and advice for future research), exploring the main contributions and implications of the study, and finally discussing the field of drama and nursing.

References

Arveklev S, Wigert H, Berg L, Lepp M (2020) Specialist nursing students' experiences of learning through drama in paediatric care. Nurse Educ Pract 43:1–6

Benedetti J (1998) Stanislavski and the actor. Methuen Drama, London

Bloom B (1956) Taxonomy of educational objectives: the classification of educational goals. Longmans, New York

Boal A (1998) Theatre of the oppressed. Pluto Press, London

de Oliveira SN, Prado MLD, Kempfer SS, Martini JG, Caravaca-Morera JA, Bernardi MC (2015) Experiential learning in nursing consultation education via clinical simulation with actors: action research. Nurse Educ Today 35(2):e50–e54

de Zulueta P (2013) Compassion in 21st century medicine: is it sustainable? Clin Ethics 8(4):119–128

Goffman E (1990) The presentation of self in everyday life. Penguin, London

Goodwin J, Deady R (2013) The art of mental health practice: the role of Drama in developing empathy. Perspect Psychiatr Care 49:126–134

Hamington M (2020) Care ethics and improvisation: can performance care? In: Stuart Fisher A, Thompson J (eds) Performing care: new perspectives on socially engaged performance. Manchester University Press, Manchester, pp 21–35

Heggestad AKT, Nortvedt P, Christiansen B, Konow-Lund A (2016) Undergraduate nursing students' ability to empathize: a qualitative study. Nurs Ethics 25(6):786–795

Hojat M (2009) Empathy in patient care: antecedents, development, measurement, and outcomes. Springer, New York

Kitson A (1987) A comparative analysis of lay-caring and professional (nursing) caring relationships. Int J Nurs Stud 24(2):155–165

Kitwood T (1997) Dementia reconsidered: the person comes first. Open University Press, Buckingham

Lawrence J, Wier J (2018) The use of drama within midwifery education to facilitate the understanding of professional behaviour and values. Midwifery 59:59–61

Lieshout F, Cardiff S (2015) Reflections on being and becoming a person-centred facilitator.
Int Pract Dev J 5. Available from: https://www.fons.org/library/journal/volume5-person-
centredness-suppl/article4. Accessed 9 Mar 2018

Macneill P, Gilmer J, Tan CH, Samarasekera DD (2016) Enhancing doctors' and healthcare professionals' patient-care role through actor-training: workshop participants' responses. Ann Acad
Med 45(5):205–211

McCormack B, McCance T (2010) Person-centred nursing: theory and practice. Wiley-Blackwell,
Chichester

Merlin B (2014) The complete Stanislavski toolkit. Nick Hern, New York

Nolan C (2009) Agency and embodiment: performing gestures/producing cultures. Harvard
University Press, Harvard

Preston S (2016) Applied theatre: facilitation: pedagogies, practices, resistance. Bloomsbury
Methuen, London

Schön DA (1983) The reflective practitioner: how professionals think in action. Basic Books,
New York

Stanislavski C (1990) An actor's handbook. Methuen, London

Conclusion, Advocating for the Dyad

9

Introduction

My doctoral study was purposefully designed with an openness at its core. I deliberately chose research questions that asked *how* applied drama can enhance person-centred nursing as an open approach to investigation. This means that any 'answers' I have presented in this book move away from affirmation or rejection. Rather, they are imprints on a path. Some of my main aims in this project have been to explore, understand, and discover if there is a potential relation between drama-based approaches to learning and the development of practical skills in PCN—specifically the PCNF process of sympathetic presence. I have been steadfast in approaching this task with an interdisciplinary mindset, which proactively seeks to differentiate between the disciplines whilst translating across them to find shared and divergent languages and approaches. As something of a novel idea, with few established texts and approaches, this book has had to break some new ground. Often, my work has had to forge an unknown path.

This final chapter is my attempt to retrace this path and articulate the patterns left behind from my journey. As a result, this final chapter will present the main contributions and implications of the study from two perspectives. The first is a specific viewpoint, where the key concepts raised throughout the study are matched against the findings of the primary research. These are the paths I planned (or rather hoped) to tread, ones where there were existing outlines and footsteps to follow. This includes those carved out by the conceptual framing in Part 1 of this book as a precursor to the primary research which was my applied ethnographic doctoral research study involving the designing and delivery of a bespoke drama-based course for nursing students. The second is a general position, an aerial view, allowing tangential and unexpected outcomes to be presented alongside the specific ones, like tributaries spanning from the central thoroughfares tracked by my research.

© The Author(s), under exclusive license to Springer Nature
Switzerland AG 2024

K. Tizzard-Kleister, *Applied Drama and Person-Centred Nursing*,
https://doi.org/10.1007/978-3-031-77208-5_9

Tracing the Path of my Journey

I wish to start this chapter by sharing an experience I had whilst undertaking my research which I explored using performance practice. I am sharing it as I believe it is analogous to the metaphor of creating pathways that represent the imprint of my doctoral study as described above. In the middle of my doctoral studies, I suffered a severe wrist injury whilst playing a contact sport. This led me to have an acute and sudden experience of my potential debility as a recipient of professional health care, particularly as my injury required surgery. I often joke that this was accidental and compulsory fieldwork. As a researcher engaged in a study exploring how drama might enhance person-centred nursing education through the concept of sympathetic presence, I found myself highly aware of how healthcare professionals interacted with me, my fellow patients, each other, and the family and friends who visited me. As a person-centred researcher, I argue it is vital to bring 'me' into my research. As explored in previous chapters, my personhood has shaped this project, I maintain my argument that it is impossible for this not to happen. As such, I felt that my experience of injury and subsequent care needed to be included in the research in some way. Likewise, as a performer I felt compelled to attend to my experience, to re-embody it, to creatively and critically explore it, and in some ways, to perform it. Over a few months, I made regular visits to the studio, to practice and play with elements of my experiences of healthcare and injury. Over that time I explored so many different aspects of my experience, many of them surprising, and some of them personally and professionally revelatory. This included, for example; the impact of one poorly put phrase in a care experience, how the memory of trauma can be unlocked through embodiment, how objects and tasks amplify and stultify interactions in clinical environments, what it feels like to experience sympathetic presence, and its absence. A crucial lesson I learnt is that it does not matter what role you have in health—every *person* has a part to play.

Along with exploring my approach to performance practice, I incorporated aspects of performative auto-ethnography in my approach. In one session, I decided to spend time to re-embody and re-perform the moment I was injured. I did this by beginning at a standing start, and then tracing a physical path with my body through space, replicating the journey I took up to, during, and just after the moment my injury occurred. I would stand ready, accelerate forward and retread the path my body took as I ran. I then focused on the collision that instigated the injury, letting my body react as if it happened again (of course, with less severity!), then slowly twisted through the air, found the moment my wrist contacted the floor, and followed through into how the rest of my body followed and came to 'rest' in the moments after. Initially, I performed this in slow motion for safety. Later I realised that my memory of this event was almost completely absent. As I repeated it, I began to gradually re-construct the experience and crucially found new access to the memories, feelings, and experience I had during my actual injury. Re-performing it over and over gave me time to think and be in that moment, in a variety of modalities. It was confronting and difficult, and sometimes cathartic. I did this for roughly 2 hours in one session. At times it was monotonous, at times meaningful. An abiding feeling I sensed was that of 'tracing a path', not just physically in the space with my body, but a renewed path for my memory, to retrace the edges of my original experience. In response to this session, I wrote, I thought, and I felt. I produced a small collage, titled 'Trace the path', which I gladly share (Fig. 9.1).

By overlaying text from this experience to the X-ray of my injury, I am creating a new path on the image. Just as I am quite literally using my finger to trace a new line on the scar from my surgery as I type this sentence. This process felt like a cathartic retracing of my experience. I do not share this to suggest high artistic

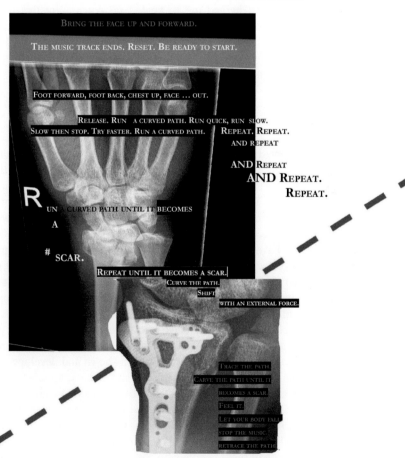

Fig. 9.1 Tracing the path, Karl Tizzard-Kleister

merit, a universality of experience for everyone, insight into a process of performance as a healing therapy, a powerful and pithy point, or even a new research method. I am sharing it because it speaks to me, giving an insight into the metaphor of tracing paths that I feel characterise my research journey. I am sharing it because I feel I cannot separate it from my research. For me, it is a powerful and sensuously embodied experience of healthcare, including nursing, and an insight into how being cared for *feels*. As well as exploring these retraced experiences in the studio, I have incorporated elements of performative auto-ethnographic practice in my teaching and when presenting my research. Through doing this I have learnt more about the power of embodied experience and developed a deeper grasp of the language of sensation, both aspects of drama that this study has highlighted as useful and relevant for person-centred nursing education.

As I touch my scar, just as when I retraced my steps into injury, I feel I am touching the limit between me now and the me who needed care at that moment. Most relevant to this study I feel as though I am touching the ethereal and temporally relocated hands of those that helped me to heal. I do not present this here as 'research' per se, but as a window into my personhood, and that liminal line separating me from health and hurt. A line we all step upon like a tightrope through our lives. Nurses, I will argue until my dying breath, are the people who most effectively bring us balance on that path.

Summary

My research study presented in this book successfully engaged a group of voluntary participants in a drama-based intervention to explore concepts raised in the literature and developed through the theoretical stages of the study. At every turn, this has been a journey of discovery. This has produced a unique, rich, and resonant approach which speaks to both research 'languages' in a meaningful way. A central concern throughout the project has been how the research can find novelty within both fields. In engaging with this, I have gained some invaluable insights into the assumptions and standard positions of each area. For instance, what might be accepted first position knowledge in one field might be radical when applied to the other. Recognising this has not been an individual process, I have often found myself relying on the expertise of others to fill my sizable gaps in knowledge. I am lucky that I have had supervisors, mentors, colleagues, and friends who have supported me and given their time with grace and generosity. I would argue that the idea of generosity describes much within this study. Generosity has been shown and developed in so many ways. Be that the generosity of my wonderful supervisors, my doctoral candidate peers, my partner whose capacity for generosity always astounds me, my family, staff from nursing and drama, attendees, and friends I have met at various research conferences, and most importantly the generosity of the participants who contributed so beautifully to this research. This research might have my name at the head, but it belongs to each of these people who have offered their time and knowledge with generosity and care.

I imagine the reader may be thinking that this sounds more suited to an acknowledgements section—and you may be right. Though I will never apologise for taking the chance to give recognition to those who thoroughly deserve it, I also argue that a significant part of the learning in this study is based on the ideas—and acts—of generosity and care. On reflection, this is an example of an aesthetic of care in action and a research project underpinned by person-centred principles. This study is the result of collaboration and interdependence. The learning in this project which has been most effective are those moments which have helped to shine a little light on how we can better engage with others by working together. This includes all of those people mentioned earlier, who have unselfishly supported me. The process of bringing two fields together to achieve this has been a privilege. Although this book represents the study to the best of my ability, a book can never capture the wealth of experiences and relationships which have served as a piece of research, this short piece has been my attempt to speak to that.

This chapter seeks to summarise the arguments and discoveries I have presented throughout this book. First, the contributions of this study to the field of knowledge will be articulated. This will be done in two parts: 'specific' and 'general' contributions. Afterwards, the implications of these contributions will be explained, again in two sections 'specific' and 'general' implications. This is important in the case of research implications emerging from this study, as it will articulate specific outcomes which point towards more focused areas for further development or implementation concerning the aims of the research, whilst the general implications serve as suggestions for wider directions of future research based on the findings of this study. The penultimate part of this final chapter will focus on the limitations of the study, outlining areas which in hindsight could benefit from a different approach and aspects of the study which could be taken on and enhanced for future research. Suggestions for future research and practice conclude this chapter.

Contributions

Summarising the richness of the findings from this study is difficult. Neither my nor the participants' experiences of this project are truly reducible to a set of four main themes, or a set of sentences representing the novel findings from this study. The question and objectives of this study were left purposefully open, to explore what might emerge naturally from the collaboration. This is important to remember when considering how the data analysis process drastically reduces, merges, and collates a variety of different findings to represent the findings of the data succinctly. In some ways, presenting the novelty in the findings of this project is difficult to do in words, seeing as much of the learning and discovery happened in the presence of others, often without words. Moreover, presenting a finding suggests the existence of a definite or exclusive answer or singular new piece of knowledge in the context of this study. From my experience and immersion in this research, I do not believe one exists in this situation. I see these distillations as potentialities rather than definitive directions. However, it is important to try and articulate these findings as clearly as possible.

I will discuss the contributions and implications in the context of each field—PCN and applied drama—but I resist the urge to separate them further. I am vehement in my belief that it is through the conjunction of the fields that the contributions were made possible in the first place. This hints at the interdependence of approaches encouraged by my interdisciplinary work. As such separating them to focus on one or the other more distinctly would undermine the ethos of this study. In short, the richness of the study is because of the bringing together of the two disciplines, separating them might make things clearer, but would severely weaken the potential impact and the specificity of the outcome in terms of interdisciplinary practice.

Specific

The first of the specific contributions offered by this study is related to how sympathetic presence can be considered performatively. Understanding sympathetic presence in this way means that it is not a trait within a singular person but is something to be felt with—and in the presence of—others. What the findings of this study contribute is a way to understand sympathetic presence in more depth and clarity than previously offered. I argue that the terminology related to sympathetic presence is vitally important in reflecting this. For instance, though using terms such as 'having', 'showing', and 'being' are satisfactory for introducing and describing the concept, it is better defined through performative terms. Sympathetic presence has often been framed as a trait—i.e., as someone having it or not. Seeing it performatively solidifies the concept and practice of sympathetic presence as an interpersonal process—as it is rightly identified as in the PCNF.

Sympathetic presence is not simply 'a performance', but a particular performative process. To perform it well it needs to be dramatically realised and practiced. Moreover, performing sympathetic presence means personhood is co-constructed in any given moment in a process of constant dialogue between the presence of everyone involved in an interaction. It is also crucial for the person-centred nurse to see that understanding sympathetic presence in this way creates conscious feedback between oneself and others—similar to how Fischer-Lichte (2008) describes how audiences and performers create a co-constructed 'auto-poetic feedback loop' during performances. Understanding this gives the person-centred nurse an approach to better understand how their presence affects others, how the presence of others affects them, and how sympathetic presence is active, not passive. Moreover, we can see how it involves a generous engagement through a dialogue between presences.

The next specific contribution is emphasising how essential sympathetic presence is to the rest of the PCN processes. Sympathetic presence is the process which best describes the immediate moment of encounter with others (or even as an intrapersonal dialogue between one and one's sense of self). It is through and within this moment that the remaining processes—working with the patient's values and beliefs, shared decision-making, engagement, and providing holistic care

(McCormack and McCance 2010)—are made possible, or begin. As described in Part 1, engagement and sympathetic presence might share a deeper affinity than previously theorised. As the findings of this study highlight, feeling sympathetic presence is in some ways symbiotic with a generosity of engagement. The more the participants engaged with the drama course and simulations with openness and commitment the more they described being able to feel sympathetic presence. The reverse is also true, where they found it easier to engage generously when they felt sympathetic presence in an interaction.

This study contributes that sympathetic presence can and should be considered as a first position to approaching interactions, which thereby enhances the other PCNF processes. Actively performing sympathetic presence means one can identify values and beliefs within others, sensitively paying attention to and working with these as they pertain to that given moment and interaction. This is also beneficial for the applied drama facilitator and intriguingly as a process for actor training. The responsiveness of the performance of sympathetic presence allows how another person is presenting themselves to affect one's approach—lighting a clearer path to making mutual decisions. How sympathetic presence is almost exclusively an embodied and experiential performance of presence gives the 'performer' access to a wealth of information on others, enhancing their ability to recognise holistic needs beyond illness or harm. More so, sympathetic presence may be a route to creating more person-centred environments, evidenced by the groups' ability to create, feel, and sustain a sense of sympathetic presence in an environment. It may be that sympathetic presence is a way to link the different 'levels' of the PCNF and a robust approach through which to 'create' a culture with a group of people.

This particular element of the contribution of this study highlights how understanding another person through sympathetic presence involves both cognitive and affective elements. Through sympathetic presence we know others by better recognising how they think and their point of view, as well as being able to engage in a non-verbal dialogue with a presence that adapts to what someone else presents. This discovery also contributes to an understanding of how sympathetic presence might help us to *be* with others as an active process and subsequently enhance how we interact with them. This is not just for PCN. This discovery reflects how sympathetic presence can be used in actor training and applied drama to access an aesthetic based on sympathy and care. This study is not positioned to offer how this might happen, or what this might look like for performance practice. However, the study certainly contributes that sympathetic presence offers a unique and affective approach to performance practices so they might be characterised by an aesthetic of care. As previously in this book, I echo Thompson (2015) and Dwyer et al. (2014) in a critique of participatory performance that focuses on cheap shock and risk as *risque*. Sympathetic presence offers a performance process and mode that mitigates against participation that is needlessly uncaring.

When considering sympathetic presence performatively, it not only 'weaves together other person-centred processes' (McCormack and McCance 2010: p. 103), it activates and enhances them. This is an important contribution to PCN research and practice, highlighting how sympathetic presence may be a direct path to person-centredness. How this relates to the applied drama field is clear and directly related to the above. Sympathetic presence offers an alternative perspective from empathy which we might encourage through applied drama facilitation. Doing so has the potential to help the field reconsider how facilitators may manage their own and their participants' emotional labour and ability to interact with others, particularly in the dilemmatic space applied drama necessarily sits within (Preston 2016). Likewise, adopting sympathetic presence could offer actor training practices a unique viewpoint on Stanislavski's MoPA and other associated approaches. My study does not offer what that might look like, but I am intrigued by the potential to bridge the divide between traditional naturalistic acting, and the theatres of practitioners like Brecht, Boal, and others. Seeing sympathetic presence as performative and relational also aligns the practice with aesthetic forms, and this study suggests that sympathetic presence can be seen as an aesthetic of care we can perform. What this means is that the educational practices of drama are uniquely well suited to enhance the skill of performing sympathetic presence. The contribution to the field of applied drama made by this study is confirmation that the approaches are transferable to PCN education, and indeed benefit from being entwined for the greatest effect. I suggest that other areas of study might benefit from the heady mix of conceptuality and embodiment that drama offers, particularly those that rely on encounters with other people. Through the performance of sympathetic presence, we can do this as a person-centred facilitator.

The last of the specific contributions is how the drama-based activity in my course seemed particularly well suited to identifying and training sympathetic presence alongside related PCN processes and concepts. Engaging in drama can be described as an aesthetic experience. It was clear that sympathetic presence was difficult for the participants to describe in words throughout the intervention. For them, it was far easier to feel, and it was certainly clearly observable when they performed it. Much of the training processes and activities in drama in a broad sense seek to engage with sensations and feelings to better prepare one for performance. This study contributes to a suggestion that drama-based approaches make it easier for PCN students to identify sympathetic presence, but also develop their ability to perform it. This is even more so in the actor training approaches used in the intervention.

The actor training approaches of Stanislavski task actors with opening themselves to their feelings and consciousness and deepening their attention to others to enhance their ability to embody them in a role. As he beautifully puts it, you must 'raise your own creative temperature' (Stanislavski 1990: p. 27), whilst being able to engage intellectually with the role you wish to perform. The skills he suggests present an easily taught and effective approach to being present in a consciously performed role which one may gear towards sympathetic presence. For example, through 'actions' one may access the psychic and 'physical life of a role' (Ibid: p. 8) you wish to consciously perform. Meanwhile, through understanding 'objectives' one can recognise and actively present the 'spiritual and physical life of *the person you are*' (Ibid: p. 149–50, emphasis added). Furthermore, there is a seemingly untapped potential for the use of the MoPA alongside other applied drama methods like Forum Theatre in far wider contexts. The contribution this study provides is that using the MoPA with other applied drama practices provides a framework through which to understand, practice, and develop communication and interaction in specific and robust ways. This study then contributes a potential route for applied drama practitioners to use to explore communication skills with the MoPA as its framework in an overwhelming variety of different contexts.

General

The initial general and less expected contribution was how the course seemed to increase confidence, whilst reducing fear and anxiety. The approach used in the research intervention seemed to give some participants the confidence to take part in further activities that they might not have taken part in otherwise, as well as feel more confident with their degree. The drama-based approach increased the participant's confidence in dealing with difficult interactive situations in the future. Engaging in the drama course promoted awareness of how the participants felt about themselves and served as a medium through which to explore personal fears and anxieties. My study contributes that acknowledging these feelings and perceptions and dealing with them transparently—particularly through interactive practical drama-based activities—increases confidence and self-awareness. Drama offered the nursing students an embodied experience, where they engaged with the language of the sensible (Berardi 2015). In this way, they did not separate theory from practice or thought from feeling.

The next general contribution was how the course seemed to increase the participants' comfort with being vulnerable and with taking what felt to them like emotional risks. Similar to how fear and anxiety were openly acknowledged and explored without judgement, the same can be said for feeling vulnerable. Following the theorisation in Chap. 3, the harm caused by intrinsically linking perceptions of risk, vulnerability, danger, and uncertainty was challenged throughout the course. The outcome shows how engaging in a drama-based course helped the participants to form a nuanced recognition of the necessity to feel and experience emotions and sometimes difficult feelings whilst working as a nurse.

The last of the identified general contributions of the study is the strong potential for the approach to enhance behaviours in practice learning experiences, and hopefully in professional practice. The direct link between the learning in the drama course to how the participants reportedly behaved whilst on practice learning placements was easily the most surprising contribution of the study. Although this link is not verified in an objective or observed sense, the impression the intervention left on how the participants considered their interactions with others when working in healthcare settings was clear and hugely encouraging. The approach directly contributed to enhanced ethical decision-making in a variety of interactive situations for the participants in practice learning. It also showed an enhanced ability to reflect on occurrences, enhanced attention to specific interpersonal details, and finer awareness of emotions in others. It remains to be seen whether colleagues and patients notice this change in the participants, but the evidence pointing to the participants' increased awareness and action on this is encouraging and certainly an intriguing area to follow up in the future.

Implications

As with the contributions of this study, the implications identified are presented in two ways: specific implications, and general implications. These implications do not intend to present a singular course of action, or indeed a singular interpretation of what the contributions of the study mean to the fields of drama and nursing. These are implications which I feel are most appropriate in light of the context and contribution of the study. In short, these are suggestions rather than directions.

It is important to consider the effect of research contributions on the field of nursing. Many argue 'that patient experience of compassionate care is […] the best measure of the nursing contribution to outcomes' (McCance and Wilson 2015: p. 1; Griffiths et al. 2008). However, that is difficult to measure for this study and many others like it. From a drama-based viewpoint, fewer implications from my study are novel. Some are distinct, such as the key implication that the notion of sympathetic presence is an alternative to empathy in practice, and indeed the concept of person-centredness as a way of understanding others can offer new ways to create and share applied drama practice. The implications are intended to be presented as a synergy between drama and nursing, to reflect the interdisciplinary nature of the project. Each implication is paired with a recommendation or a suggestion for a future direction. These implications broadly focus on the areas of education, research, and practice.

Specific

The first of the identified specific implications is in response to how the findings suggest that sympathetic presence happens between people. This implies that as sympathetic presence is a fundamentally embodied experience, it is easier to be felt and experienced than explained verbally or cognitively. Furthermore, this implies that how sympathetic presence has been identified and assessed needs to be re-evaluated. It is recommended that drama-based approaches be integrated into education and assessment situations to enhance the student's and the tutor's ability to recognise sympathetic presence. It is implied and recommended that drama-based approaches offer a practical framework for developing an ability to feel, assess, and perform sympathetic presence. In terms of research, this implies that methods of examining sympathetic presence as a phenomenon may be best served by integrating experiential accounts alongside more objective and/or observational measures. This will help to ensure that both the observable and experiential sensations associated with sympathetic presence are accounted for in research studies. How this implication relates to practice is fairly clear, when interacting with others one must be conscious of one's embodied presence to perform sympathetic presence. What emerges as a further implication to this is the potential strategic use of simulation and role play in education to scaffold between practice learning and aid PCN development in students, and the clear path this work has towards enhancing interactive capabilities. How this study has adapted SRP, in particular applying the MoPA within a space of potentiality through applied drama practice, implies how much there is to gain from adopting interdisciplinarity which privileges the expertise of each discipline in SRP and associated practices.

The next specific implication is based on the findings that highlighted the potential enhancements in interpersonal skills as a result of taking part in a drama-based activity. This finding implies that though there is ample evidence that drama-based approaches applied to PCN education enhance communication, there is more work to be done to specify and objectively assess these enhancements. As a result, educational approaches should be reconsidered to make use of this potential. It is recommended that future research projects focus on specific features of interpersonal skills with other PCN processes. One example would be how non-verbal communication and engagement may be enhanced through a drama-based approach. The implication relies on the reflection of the participants and my observation of them. It is therefore also recommended to explore this potential outcome in other ways, including adding objective empirical measures alongside the types of data in this study.

In terms of practice, these skills offer an easily adaptable and usable interactive approach for PCN in a variety of situations. Applying this approach in practice is recommended yet implies–again—further study on this practical application. The implication here is that applied drama adopts wider forms of research more readily, not just to appease a perceived need from other disciplines or funders, but to grow an evidence base that captures the breadth and depth of the practice and application of drama approaches to areas like PCN. Mirroring this, there is an implication that sympathetic presence has great potential as a theoretical and practical approach to accessing an aesthetic of care within performance practices. It certainly adds to the vocabulary of the aesthetics of care as a relational and performative practice.

The last specific implication is that a drama-based approach might be applied in more depth to educational PCN settings. It is recommended that the approach becomes integrated into the existing nursing curriculum in a robust and meaningful way. The findings from this study point towards the potential richness that the interdisciplinary approach would have for first-year PCN students, and I would expect this to be true for second- and third-year students also. The implication arising from this is that any integration of the approach should be introduced early and sustained strategically to practice learning experiences throughout the nursing degree. More research could be conducted to ascertain how these effects are manifest during practice learning and beyond. What this suggests as a further implication is that using pedagogy from drama can offer ways to improve simulation practice, and to better bridge the gap between theory and practice for nursing students.

General

The first of the two general implications of the study suggests following up on and strengthening the identified findings in more detail in future research. These include the findings which suggest improved confidence, reduced anxiety, readiness to be vulnerable and take emotional risks, and encouragement of ethical action in practice learning, amongst more. Educationally the potential is intriguing and implies that discovering whether these outcomes are more generalisable is a fruitful direction for future travel. The recommendation is that each facet could be explored in its own right with a suitable research study, potentially focused again in an educational setting. As mentioned, this study always intended to light the path towards more specific areas for future study, as well as how this might affect outcomes for PCN in practice. The above represents the key areas identified through the study that could be explored in more depth. What seems to be clear to me at this stage is that engaging in the creative arts and in particular participating through drama pedagogy is synergistic with person-centred nursing and many of its values.

The second general implication suggests taking the approach into different contexts to discover whether these are generalisable outcomes shared across various areas such as in clinical practice, in community settings, mental health settings, at management levels, and so on. The findings of this study are contextual, relying on subjective and specific sources of data and interpretation. Though this adds to the richness of the findings, it cannot be ignored that this implies that a similar experience might not necessarily be shared by other groups in different contexts. The recommendation here is to explore ways in which this approach can be applied and adapted for different contexts. The implication is that though drama-based approaches worked in the ways that they did in this context with this particular group of people, more needs to be done to test the transferability of these outcomes. This includes looking at areas beyond PCN, such as medical education, social work, community nursing, midwifery, and so on. As identified in this book, many projects exist across the world, each using drama in fairly unique ways to enhance healthcare education. I argue this study provides clear evidence that applying drama into healthcare creates invigorating educational spaces, where students can be challenged, learn about themselves and others, find better ways to be active agents in the world, and so much more in a safe and supportive environment. I speculate that the approach I have taken is transferable, and if conducted with the same facilitative approach should produce similar outcomes in a wide variety of settings and contexts. A strength of the transferability of drama approaches is seeing drama as a methodology of learning and practice, meaning that the 'content' and 'concept' can be taken up from the discipline it is being applied to. This requires expertise in applied drama theory and practice to manage successfully. I therefore add an argument I hope will endure as an implication from my research, that interdisciplinary work is best conducted by a dyad, in this case, a pair of people who work together across their differences for a shared purpose, learning from one another and sharing insight that is generative and full of potentiality.

Finally, there is a particular implication for applied drama to look to other areas of drama-based activity and ways of researching with more open arms. This study has intertwined theories and practices from PCN and drama-based areas. The openness of dialogue between these approaches resulted in an interdisciplinary methodology characterised by—poignantly—sympathetic presence. By adopting this approach applied drama may welcome practical approaches like Stanislavski's MoPA, and PCN-influenced research approaches, as this study did. There is positive potential for further collaborations to explore the impact their conjunction will make. This study is a testament to the effectiveness of allowing disciplines to meet and work across divides to produce new meaning and light new and unexpected paths. Both drama and nursing have their prejudices as fields of practice and research. I have encountered some of these through my research and practice. Another abiding implication of my work will be to challenge and attempt to disrupt disciplinary territorialism. As this chapter has explained, the vibrancy of this study has been the result of generosity from many people. It is generosity that best disrupts the disciplinary divides, leading to a willingness to share and to learn that challenges your own established knowledge.

Conclusion and Suggestions for Future Research

In this chapter, I have summarised the journey I have undertaken in this piece of work and have presented the contributions and implications identified in the study. Throughout, suggestions for the next steps in work like this have been provided.

The main suggestion I make for future work is to continue with dialogic interdisciplinarity in a way that uses the best of both 'worlds' to come together to make things better and find new and unexpected ways to work. One final addition to this notion is that this can and should be done through a process characterised by sympathetic presence as a first position. In this case, drama-based approaches have been applied to PCN in educational contexts and concepts. The result was a deeper understanding of sympathetic presence through the concepts of performativity. There is vast scope for more work to find other ways that PCN and drama-based approaches might link. This study has laid the ground for a process to discover ways the two fields might speak to one another, learn from one another, and discover insights through coming together with a shared purpose. This study has advocated for interdisciplinary work as the work of a dyad. It is not so much about drama, as it is not really about nursing. It is about drama *and* nursing.

References

Berardi F (2015) And: phenomenology of the end. Semiotext(e), South Pasadena

Dwyer P, Hunter MA, Pearson JS (2014) High stakes: performance and risk. [editorial]. About Perf 12(1):1–5

Fischer-Lichte E (2008) The transformative power of performance. Routledge, London

Griffiths P, Jones S, Maben J, Murrells T (2008) State of the art metrics for nursing: a rapid appraisal. National Nursing Research Unit, King's College London, London

McCance T, Wilson V (2015) Using person-centred key performance indicators to improve paediatric services: an international ventures. Int Pract Dev J 5. Available from: https://www.fons.org/Resources/Documents/Journal/Vol5Suppl/IPDJ_05(suppl)_08.pdf. Accessed 20 Mar 2018

McCormack B, McCance T (2010) Person-Centred nursing: theory and practice. Wiley-Blackwell, Chichester

Preston S (2016) Applied theatre: facilitation: pedagogies, practices, resistance. Bloomsbury Methuen, London

Stanislavski C (1990) An actor's handbook. Methuen, London

Thompson J (2015) Towards an aesthetics of care. Res Drama Educ : The Journal of Applied Theatre and Performance 20(4):430–441

Printed in the United States
by Baker & Taylor Publisher Services